Laparoscopic Hernia Repair
How to Learn at Ease

Video Contents*

1.	Laparoscopic Anatomy of Inguinal Region		Video 1.1
2.	Different Types of Hernia Repair	▪ Inguinal—Direct and Indirect, TAPP, TEP and 2-port TEP ▪ Umbilical Hernia Repair ▪ Femoral Hernia Repair ▪ Lumbar Hernia Repair ▪ Sliding Hernia Repair	Videos 2.1 and 2.2
3.	Troubleshooting During Hernia Repair	▪ Combined Procedures ▪ Multiple Hernias ▪ Hernia with Adhesion ▪ Mesh Placement our Technique ▪ Obstructed Hernia ▪ Recurrent Hernia ▪ Strangulated Hernia	Video 3.1
4.	Innovations in Ventral Hernia Repair	▪ Sleeve with Abdominoplasty ▪ eTEP ▪ Hybrid Hernia Repair	Videos 4.1 to 4.3
5.	Unedited Videos	TEP, TAPP, Ventral Hernia Repair	Videos 5.1 to 5.7
6.	Pediatric Hernia	▪ Laparoscopic Female Hernia Repair ▪ Laparoscopic Male Hernia Repair ▪ Open Pediatric Hernia Repair by MIS	Videos 6.1 to 6.3

To access the videos online, kindly scan the QR code

**All Edited Videos Demonstrated with Voice-over.*

Laparoscopic Hernia Repair
How to Learn at Ease

Second Edition

R Padmakumar
DNB MNAMS FAIS Dip ALS FCLS FIMSA FRCS
Senior Consultant and Head
Department of Minimally Invasive Surgery
VPS Lakeshore Hospital and Keyhole Clinic
Kochi, Kerala, India

D Madhukara Pai
MS FCLS Dip MAS (Hernia) FLHS eFIAGES FISCP
Senior Consultant General and Laparoscopic Surgeon
Department of Minimally Invasive Surgery
VPS Lakeshore Hospital and Keyhole Clinic
Senior Faculty
Verwandeln Institute
Kochi, Kerala, India

Foreword
Mahesh C Misra

JAYPEE
JAYPEE BROTHERS MEDICAL PUBLISHERS
The Health Sciences Publisher
New Delhi | London

Jaypee Brothers Medical Publishers (P) Ltd

Headquarters
EMCA House
23/23-B, Ansari Road, Daryaganj
New Delhi 110 002, India
Landline: +91-11-23272143, +91-11-23272703
+91-11-23282021, +91-11-23245672
E-mail: jaypee@jaypeebrothers.com

Corporate Office
4838/24, Ansari Road, Daryaganj
New Delhi 110 002, India
Phone: +91-11-43574357
Fax: +91-11-43574314
E-mail: jaypee@jaypeebrothers.com

Overseas Office
J.P. Medical Ltd
83 Victoria Street, London
SW1H 0HW (UK)
Phone: +44 20 3170 8910
E-mail: info@jpmedpub.com

EU GPSR Authorised Representative
Logos Europe, 9 rue Nicolas Poussin
17000, La Rochelle, France
Phone: +33 (0) 6 67 93 73 78
E-mail: contact@logoseurope.eu

Website: www.jaypeebrothers.com
Website: www.jaypeedigital.com

Inquiries for bulk sales may be solicited at: jaypee@jaypeebrothers.com

Laparoscopic Hernia Repair—How to Learn at Ease

First Edition: 2017

Second Edition: 2024

Reprint: **2025**

ISBN: 978-93-5696-281-1

Printed in India

From the Authors' Desk

Repair of simple and complex abdominal hernia by laparoscopic technique is now the method of choice in most centers. Laparoscopic repair offers outcomes equivalent to open repair with the additional benefits of greater patient satisfaction and reduced hospitalization. For some hernias, notably incisional hernia and hiatal hernia, the technique appears to be superior to conventional surgery.

Open hernia surgery is usually considered a basic surgical technique while laparoscopic hernia repair is considered an advanced procedure. The reason for this is that we have been studying inguinal canal anatomy since our first year of undergraduate classes. But laparoscopic anatomy is not usually taught. It is our aim to make the procedure easy and learnable to young practicing surgeons. In this book, a detailed description of laparoscopic anatomy is given. It also gives definite guidance to patient selection and operative techniques. Each procedure is illustrated with a series of high-quality photographs in a step-by-step manner, allowing the reader to follow the sequence of the operation. The recognition and management of complications is highlighted, and postoperative management is also described. In the consecutive section, background information about hernia is detailed. This operative guide offers a complete analysis of each of the current technologies and is a valuable source of information for practitioners and trainee surgeons. In this edition, we have included eTEP, TARM, abdominoplasty, hybrid hernia repair, mesh and mesh fixations, and anatomy of transversalis fascia.

R Padmakumar
DNB MNAMS FAIS Dip ALS FCLS FIMSA FRCS
Senior Consultant and Head
+91 9447230370; 9846320370
drrpadmakumar@gmail.com

D Madhukara Pai
MS FCLS Dip MAS (Hernia) FLHS eFIAGES FISCP
Senior Consultant General and Laparoscopic Surgeon
+91 9847278663
mkarpai@gmail.com

Please log onto our websites:
www.drrpadmakumar.com
www.keyholeclinic.in

Foreword

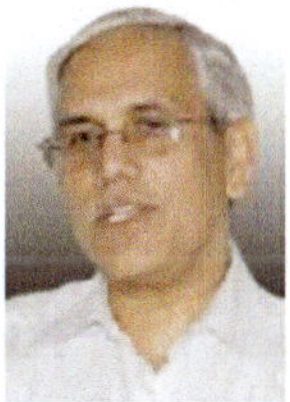

Video of laparoscopic cholecystectomy (LC) was first time viewed by surgeons in 1989 with disbelief and excitement together at the Society of American Gastrointestinal and Endoscopic Surgeons (SAGES) in USA. A German Surgeon Muhe performed first LC in 1986 and subsequently two French Surgeons—Mouret and Dubois introduced LC to the world. The procedure was adopted and accepted worldwide. Laparoscopic cholecystectomy spread like a wildfire across the globe despite higher incidence of common bile duct injury even today. Video-assisted Minimally Invasive Surgery has been termed as the unparalleled surgical revolution and we entered the Silver Jubilee year of Minimally Invasive or Minimal Access Surgery in 2014.

After cholecystectomy, the next elective general surgical procedure, which is performed by every general surgeon, is groin hernia repair. Every general surgical trainee starts his or her surgical debut with an open hernia repair, appendectomy and then gallbladder in that order. Therefore, it is not surprising that laparoscopic cholecystectomy has been the "Gold Standard" index procedure to be taught and learnt by all surgical trainees around the world by the sheer volume of the symptomatic and/or asymptomatic gallbladder disease over the last 25 years.

Although the number of open groin hernia repairs are also performed in large numbers (700,000/year in USA) but penetration of laparoscopic groin hernia repair has been limited and rather low, not only in India, China (<4%) but even in USA, UK (around 20%) and Europe (up to 30%). As soon as we talk of laparoscopic groin hernia repair, it becomes an advanced laparoscopic procedure. There is a definite longer learning curve and rarely serious operative complications (vascular, bowel and urinary bladder), which have been unknown during open groin hernia repair. There are two standard laparoscopic techniques for the repair of groin hernia, i.e., transabdominal preperitoneal (TAPP) and totally extraperitoneal (TEP) repair over the last 25 years. There have been a large number of laparoscopic groin hernia operations performed worldwide but there are extremely limited opportunities for surgeons to get exposure and training in the two techniques.

Live operative workshops in which expert surgeons perform these procedures for the benefit of the trainees and practicing surgeons have a limited role to the extent that trainees get to know the technique and get encouraged to learn and develop into a laparoscopic hernia surgeon. I firmly believe that a surgeon, who labels himself or herself as a Laparoscopic Hernia Surgeon, must be familiar with both the techniques, i.e., TAPP and TEP for the simple reason that in case of conversion from TEP, TAPP is a fall-back procedure. The best way to teach and learn laparoscopic hernia repair or, for that matter, any laparoscopic/endoscopic procedure is by preceptorship and proctorship model, which is a quick, effective and safe way to teach and learn laparoscopic or open surgery.

This book shall help general surgeons acquire basic knowledge about the anatomical basis and surgical techniques of repair of both groin and ventral/incisional hernia and also other hernias. I have focused on laparoscopic groin hernia repair because laparoscopic ventral/incisional hernia repair is less difficult to learn and perform. I am confident that this monograph will come in handy for those surgeons, who would want to begin to learn the art and craft of laparoscopic repair of various abdominal wall defects. Going through the monograph, it seems that the most significant challenge was to have originality of illustrations, diagrams and operative pictures depicting anatomy and the steps of the procedure. I hope the authors have taken due care about the originality of their work and any of the words reproduced has been duly acknowledged. I am delighted to write a Foreword for this work produced by Dr R Padmakumar and Dr D Madhukara Pai on *Laparoscopic Hernia Repair—How to Learn at Ease.*

Mahesh C Misra
MBBS MS FRCS (Glasgow) FAMS (India) FACS (USA) FCLS (India)
Hon FRCS (Glasgow) DSc (Hon Causa) Hon FRCS (Edinburgh)
Emeritus Professor
JPN Apex Trauma Center
All India Institute of Medical Sciences
Program and Course Director, ATLS India Program
Former Professor (General and Minimally Invasive Surgery)
Former Director of Surgical Disciplines
Former President and Vice Chancellor
Mahatma Gandhi University of Medical Sciences and Technology
Jaipur, Rajasthan, India
mcmisra@gmail.com

Acknowledgments

We express our gratitude to the people who helped get our dream materialized.

We are obliged to Mrs Premna Subin, Mr Subin Thomas and Mrs Renu Reghunath for editorial assistance.

We express our sincere thanks to Dr Farish Shamsudeen, Dr Kumar Abhishek, Mr Subin Thomas, and Mr Sreenath for the drawings and pictures.

We are grateful to all our colleague doctors, especially, Dr Resen Rajan, Dr Karthik K (Anesthesiologists), OPD staff, Keyhole Clinic team, theater nurses, floor staff and paramedical staff for all their efforts in taking care of our patients in an excellent manner.

We express our gratitude to our teachers and family members, who always gave us their support.

We are grateful to all our trainees and our patients, who raised us to this level to make the project happen.

We place on record our sincere gratitude to the office bearers of Indian Hernia Society, especially Professor Dr MC Misra for the invaluable encouragement. Our heartfelt gratitude to the office bearers and members of the Association Surgeons of India for the support in all over endeavors.

We express our gratitude to the office bearers of SELSI (Society of Endoscopic and Laparoscopic Surgeons of India.

We especially appreciate the constant support and encouragement of Shri Jitendar P Vij (Group Chairman) and Mr Ankit Vij (Managing Director) of M/s Jaypee Brothers Medical Publishers (P) Ltd, New Delhi, India, in publishing the book and also their associates, particularly Ms Chetna Malhotra (Senior Director—Professional Publishing, Marketing, and Business Development), and Ms Charu Lata (Development Editor), who have been prompt, efficient, and most helpful.

Contents

Chapter

1 Introduction to Hernia Repair

INTRODUCTION

Repair of inguinal hernia is one of the most common surgical procedures performed worldwide. The lifetime risk for men is 27% and for women, it is 3%.[1]

"No disease of the human body, belonging to the province of the surgeon, requires in its treatment, a better combination of accurate, anatomical knowledge with surgical skill than hernia in all its variants."

—Sir Astley Paston Cooper (Fig. 1),
The Anatomy and Surgical Treatment of Inguinal and Congenital Hernia,
Cox, London, 1804

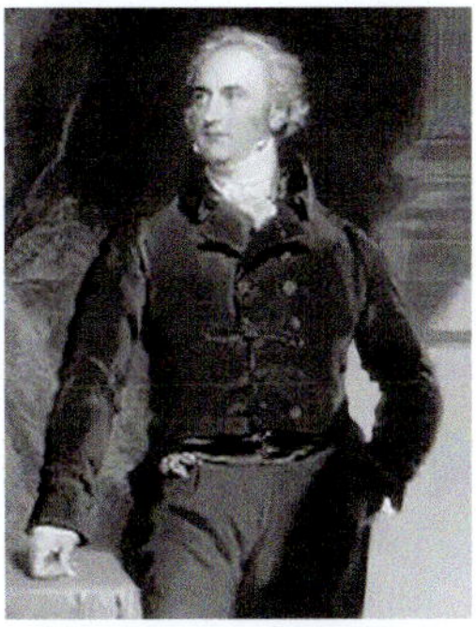

Fig. 1: Sir Astley Paston Cooper.

"I know more than hundred surgeons whom I would cheerfully allow to remove my gallbladder but only one to whom I should like to expose my inguinal canal."

—Sir Henage Ogilvie (Fig. 2)

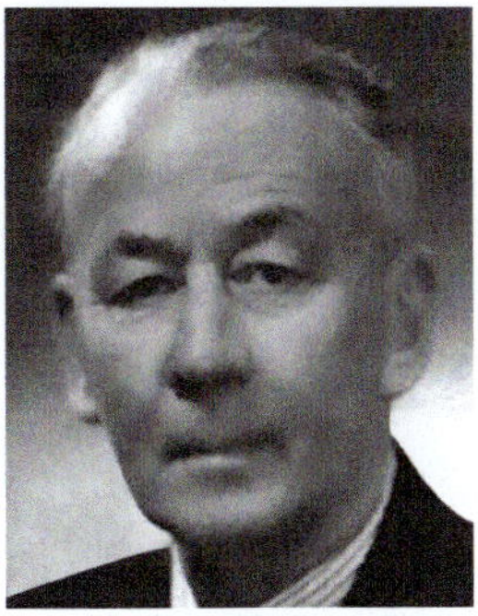

Fig. 2: Sir Henage Ogilvie.

REFERENCE

1. Primatesta P, Goldacre MJ. Inguinal hernia repair: Incidence of elective and emergency surgery, readmission, and mortality. Int J Epidemiol. 1996;25:835-9.

Chapter

2 History of Hernia Repair

Year	*Proponent*	*Procedure details*[1]	
1884	Edoardo Bassini	Introduced the modern era of herniorrhaphy. Bassini's method relies on a musculoaponeurotic repair to reconstruct the inguinal canal	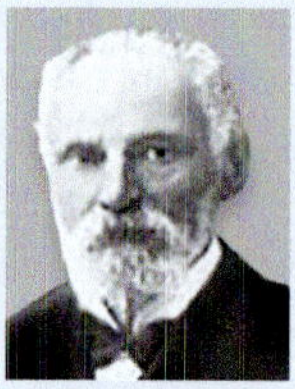 Edoardo Bassini
1945	Edward Earle Shouldice	Four-layer repair	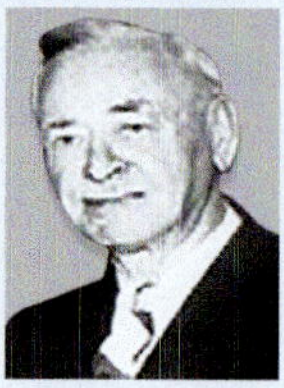 Edward Earle Shouldice
1958	Francis C. Usher	Used polypropylene as the first successful synthetic prosthesis	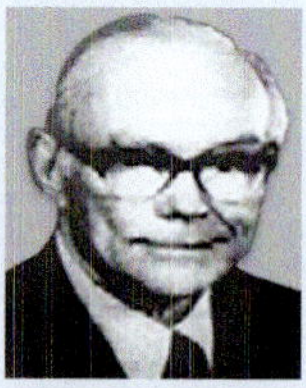 Francis C. Usher
1964	Irving L. Lichtenstein	Tension-free open mesh repair. Till now, it is the standard evidence-based operation	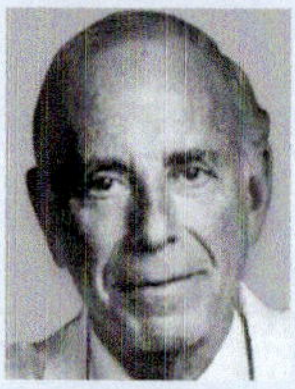 Irving L. Lichtenstein

Contd...

Contd...

Year	*Proponent*	*Procedure details*[1]	
1973	Rene Stoppa	Giant prosthetic reinforcement of visceral sac (GPRVS)/open preperitoneal mesh repair (significantly reduced recurrence rate for multirecurrent groin hernias). He reiterated the advantages of the posterior approach	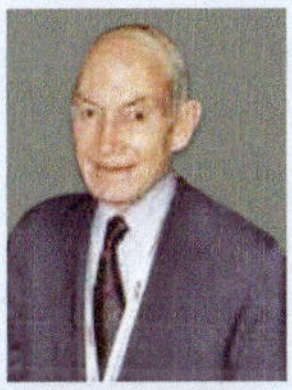 Rene Stoppa
1982	Ralph Ger	The first laparoscopic hernia repair by approximating the internal ring with stainless steel clips	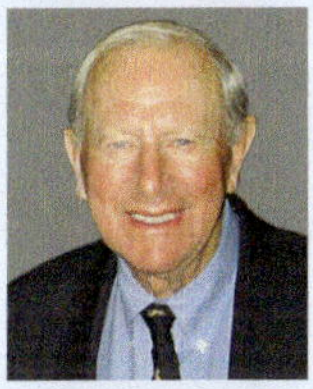 Ralph Ger
1992	Maurice E. Arregui	Transabdominal preperitoneal (TAPP) repair	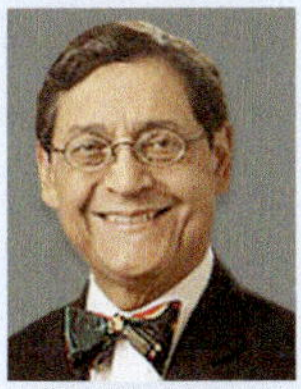 Maurice E. Arregui
1992	Yves Marie Dion	Transabdominal preperitoneal (TAPP) repair	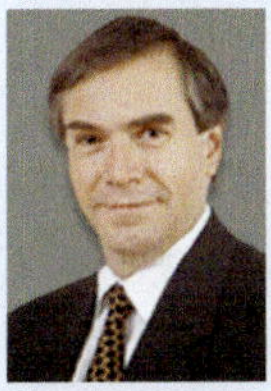 Yves Marie Dion
1992	Ferzli et al., Dulucq, Himpens, McKernan, and Laws	Totally extraperitoneal (TEP) repair	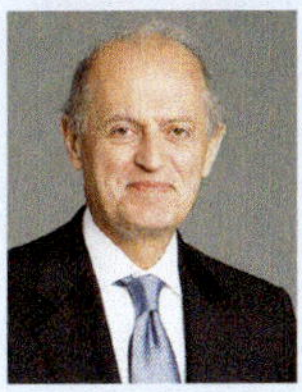 Ferzli

Pioneers in laparoscopic hernia surgery.

Both transabdominal preperitoneal (TAPP) repair and totally extraperitoneal (TEP) repair, the techniques of laparoscopic hernia repair, reproduce the concept of Stoppa, by placing a large mesh in the preperitoneal space to cover half of the abdominal wall and all the weak areas (myopectineal orifice of Fruchaud) including area of internal ring, Hasselbach's triangle, and the femoral ring with/without obturator opening. Both TAPP and TEP repair are now accepted as evidence-based treatment for inguinal hernias equivalent to Lichtenstein's procedure.

REFERENCE

1. Hee RV. History of inguinal hernia repair. Jurnalul de Chirurgie, Iaşi. 2011;7(3).

Chapter 3

Laparoscopic Hernia Repair: Advantages and Difficulties

Laparoscopic hernia repair has got definite advantages and difficulties as well. They are as follows:

ADVANTAGES[1,2]

Level 1A Evidence

- Lower incidence of wound infection and hematoma formation
- Lesser pain and discomfort; immediate postoperative pain and delayed pain are reduced
- Shorter hospital stay
- Early resumption of normal daily activities and work.

Level 1B Evidence

- Incidence of recurrence as low as Lichtenstein's repair
- Cost-effective when quality-adjusted life-year (QALY) is taken into consideration.

Level 4 Evidence

- Deep repair of inguinal hernia addresses the issue of repair at the "point of origin" rather than at the "point of presentation." This gives a mechanical advantage over the onlay/anterior mesh placement.
- Covering the entire myopectineal orifice of Fruchaud, the deep repair deals with all the potential sites at risk for herniation in the groin.
- Other coexisting diseases such as cholelithiasis can be tackled in the same sitting.
- Larger mesh can be placed comfortably when compared to that in open technique.
- Reduces the chance of infection (mesh and wound) as wound is minimal and mesh is deep inside.
- Preferred in recurrence after anterior approach as preperitoneal space is untouched and dissection is easy.

DIFFICULTIES

Level 1A Evidence

Longer operation time.

Level 2B Evidence

Steeper learning curve: A safe and successful outcome of any surgical procedure is dependent upon the clear understanding of the surgical anatomy of the relevant area. The laparoscopic view of the groin anatomy is quite different from that during open surgery. The laparoscopic view is essentially a posterior approach view. Most surgeons are well versed in the anterior approach. Changing to the laparoscopic approach needs additional knowledge. Certain structures that are clearly visible during the open approach such as the ilioinguinal nerve and the inguinal ligament are not as clearly visible with the laparoscope. It is not mandatory to visualize them as you rely on median, medial, and lateral infraumbilical ligaments, inferior epigastric vessels, pubic symphysis, pubic arch, iliopubic tract, external iliac vessels, cord structures, etc.

Level 4 Evidence

- The laparoscopic view is a "virtual view" with a "two-dimensional" handicap. There is additional loss of tactile feedback.
- Hand-eye coordination is the key as in any other laparoscopic procedure.
- The procedure may be difficult if the preperitoneal space is dissected during prior surgeries.

REFERENCES

1. Kavic SM. Laparoscopic versus open repair: a superior approach to inguinal herniorrhaphy? OA Minimally Invasive Surgery. 2013;1(1):1.
2. Simons MP, Aufenacker T, Bay-Nielsen M, Bouillot JL, Campanelli G, Conze J, et al. European Hernia Society guidelines on the treatment of inguinal hernia in adult patients. Hernia. 2009;13(4):343-403.

Chapter

4 Anatomy of Inguinal Region

THE "MYOPECTINEAL ORIFICE OF FRUCHAUD"[1-5]

All groin (inguinofemoral) hernias originate in a single weak area called the myopectineal orifice. This oval, funnel-like, "potential" orifice formed by the following structures, makes the "myopectineal orifice of Fruchaud" **(Figs. 1 and 2)**.

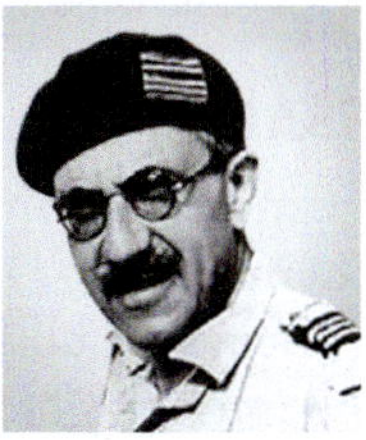

Fig. 1: Henry Fruchaud.

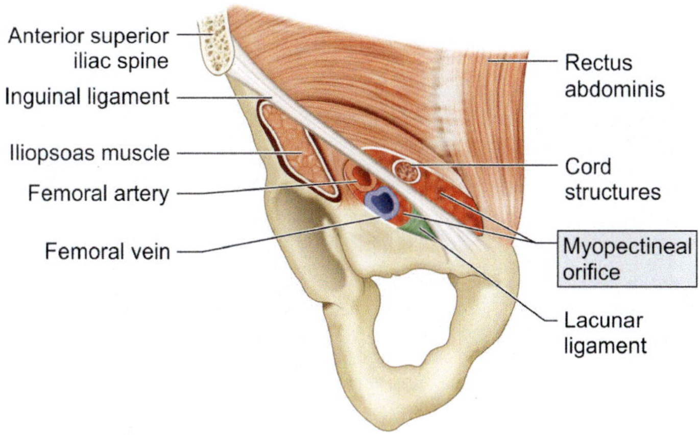

Fig. 2: Myopectineal orifice of Fruchaud.

BOUNDARIES

Superiorly	Internal oblique and transversus abdominis muscles
Inferiorly	Superior pubic ramus
Medially	Rectus muscle sheath

PERITONEAL LANDMARKS[1-5]

Median umbilical ligament: This ligament ascends in the median plane from the apex of the bladder to the umbilicus. It represents the obliterated allantoic duct and its lower part is the site of the rare urachal cyst.

Medial umbilical ligament: This ligament represents the obliterated umbilical artery on each side and can be traced down to the internal iliac artery.

Lateral umbilical ligament: It is the ridge of peritoneum, which is raised by the inferior epigastric vessels.

These ligaments delineate the infraumbilical fossae **(Fig. 3)**.

INFRAUMBILICAL FOSSAE (FIG. 4)

Infraumbilical fossae are important for surgeons due to the following reasons:

- Delineate the sites of groin herniation
- An important landmark for orientation during hernia repairs
    - *Supravesical fossae:* The infraumbilical area between the median and medial umbilical ligaments. This is the site for the origin of the supravesical hernia.

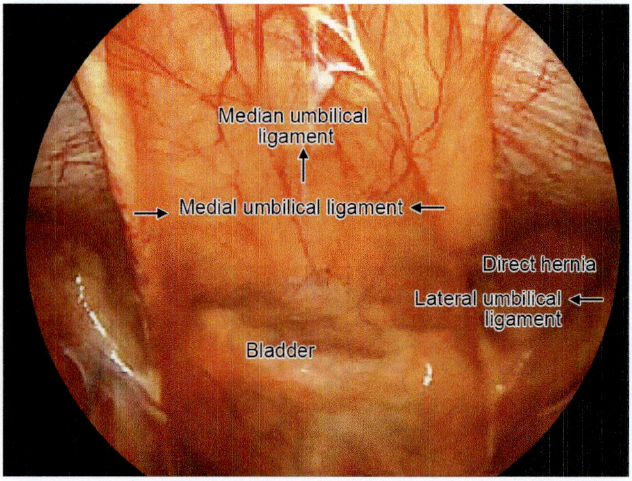

Fig. 3: Infraumbilical ligaments.

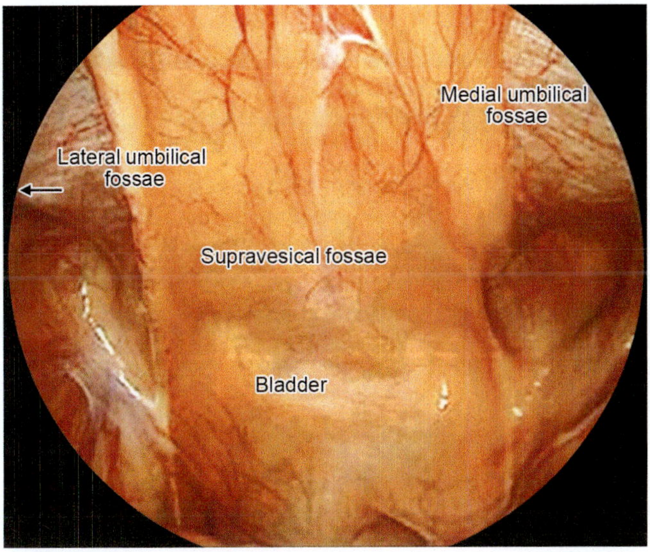

Fig. 4: Infraumbilical fossae.

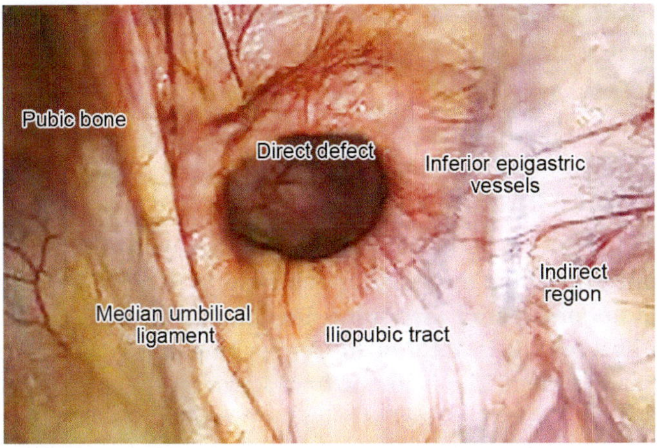

Fig. 5: Inguinal region laparoscopically.

- *Medial umbilical fossae:* The infraumbilical area between the medial and lateral umbilical ligaments. This is the site for the origin of the femoral and direct inguinal hernia **(Fig. 5)**.
- *Lateral umbilical fossae:* The infraumbilical area lateral to the lateral umbilical ligament. This is the site for the origin of the indirect inguinal hernia.

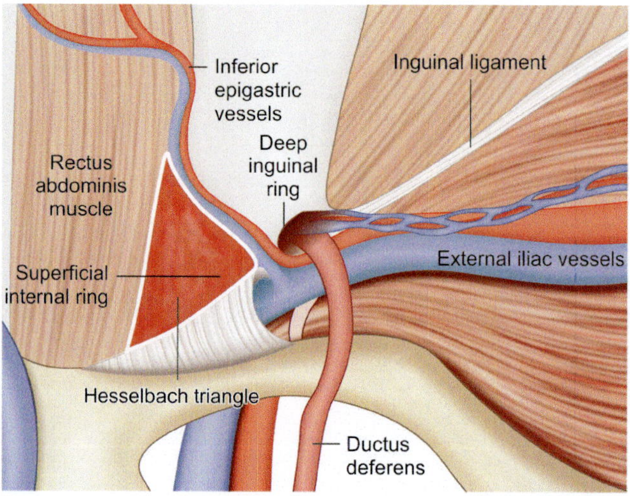

Fig. 6: Hesselbach's triangle.

Hesselbach's Triangle (by Franz Caspar Hesselbach)[1-5] (Fig. 6)

Superolateral boundary	Inferior epigastric vessels
Medial boundary	Rectus sheath
Inferior boundary	Cooper's ligament/inguinal ligament

It is the site for direct hernia.

ILIOPUBIC TRACT

The iliopubic tract is a thickened lateral extension of the transversalis fascia, which runs from the superior pubic ramus to the iliopectineal arch and the anterior superior iliac spine. It is intimately associated with the inguinal ligament. It is anterior to Cooper's ligament and posterior to the inguinal ligament. The iliopubic tract separates the internal ring from the femoral canal. It is visualized as a fibrous (white) tract.

TRANSVERSALIS FASCIA (OF GALLAUDET)[1-5]

Transversalis fascia is a two-layered structure. The anterior fatty layer is adherent to the rectus abdominis muscle. The posterior layer lies in between the preperitoneal fascia and fatty layer. It divides this space into an anterior (vascular space) and a posterior avascular preperitoneal space.

Prevesical Space of Retzius

The preperitoneal space that lies deep to the supravesical fossa, and the medial umbilical fossa is the prevesical space of Retzius (described in 1858, by Swedish anatomist Anders Retzius). This space contains loose connective tissue and fat. It extends laterally as space of Bogros over iliopsoas muscle.

Important structures in these spaces are:

- *Arteries:*
  - External iliac artery
  - Inferior epigastric artery and its branches

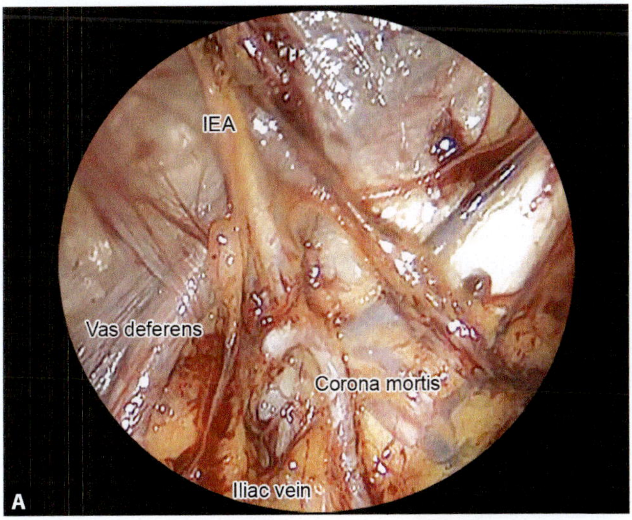

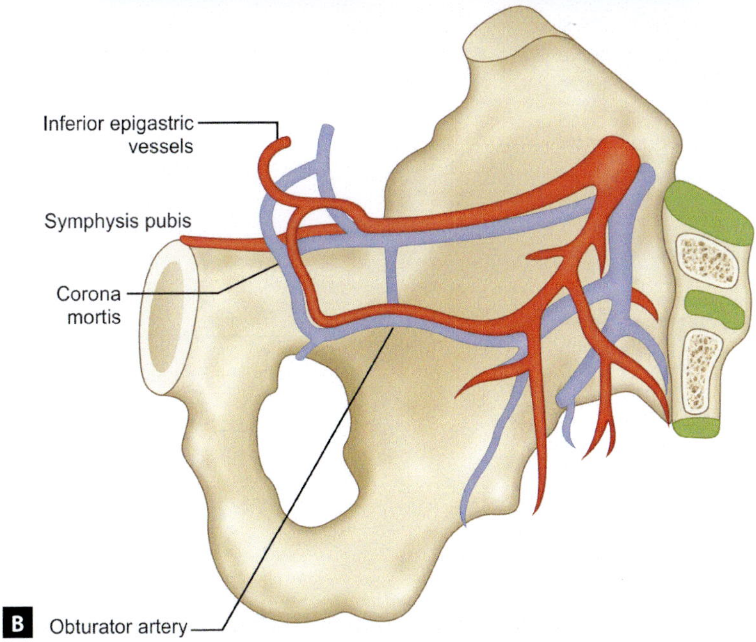

Figs. 7A and B: Corona mortis. (IEA: inferior epigastric artery)

- *Veins:*
  - External iliac vein
  - Inferior epigastric veins
  - Deep venous circulation
- *Nerves:*
  - Lateral femoral cutaneous nerve
  - Genitofemoral nerve
  - Femoral nerve
- *Lymphatics and lymph nodes*

Pubic branches: The inferior epigastric artery gives rise to the anterior pubic artery, which along with the iliopubic vein crosses the superior pubic ramus. In 25–30% of individuals, the anterior pubic branch is large and can replace the obturator artery. This large arterial branch (aberrant obturator artery) can partially encircle the neck of a hernia sac and be injured in a femoral hernia repair. It could also be injured while dissecting on to the Cooper's ligament. So, the whole anastomotic ring is known as the "corona mortis" (circle of death)[6] **(Figs. 7A and B)**.

Deep venous circulation of the preperitoneal space (Bendavid): The venous circle/deep venous circulation of Bendavid[7] is located at the subinguinal

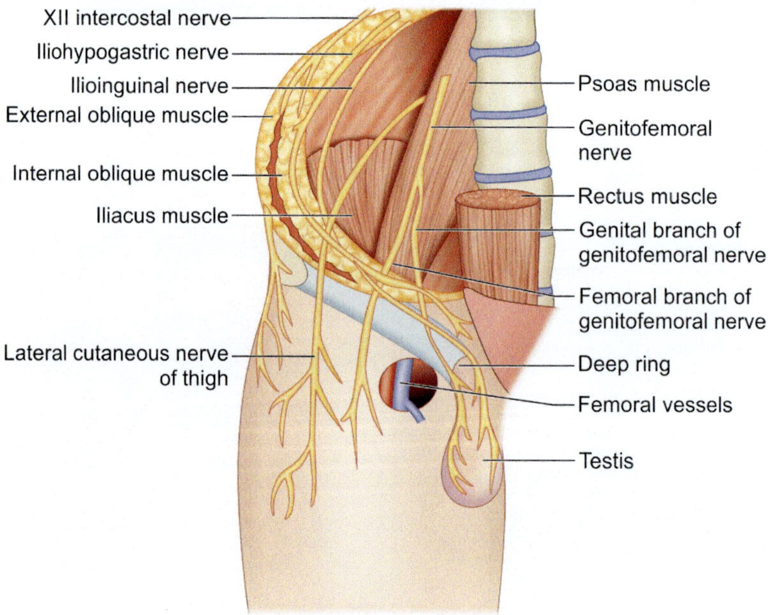

Fig. 8: Nerves in the inguinal region.

space of Bogros. It is a network of deep inferior epigastric, rectusial, and suprapubic and retropubic veins. These are important because damage to these vessels is easy and usually leads to hematoma formation.

Nerves in the inguinal region[8-10] **(Fig. 8)**:

The following three nerves are at risk for injury during dissection:

1. Lateral femoral cutaneous nerve
2. Femoral branch of genitofemoral nerve
3. Obturator nerve

The following nerves are usually not at risk during dissection but can be injured if excessive pressure is applied during mesh fixation:

- Ilioinguinal nerve
- Iliohypogastric nerve
- Genital branch of genitofemoral nerve.

INGUINAL ANATOMY WITH THE PERITONEUM INTACT[11] (FIG. 9)

With the introduction of the laparoscope into the abdomen, five important landmarks can be identified in the infraumbilical region:

1. Inferior epigastric vessels
2. Medial umbilical ligament
3. Spermatic vessels
4. Vas deferens
5. Trapezoid of disaster.

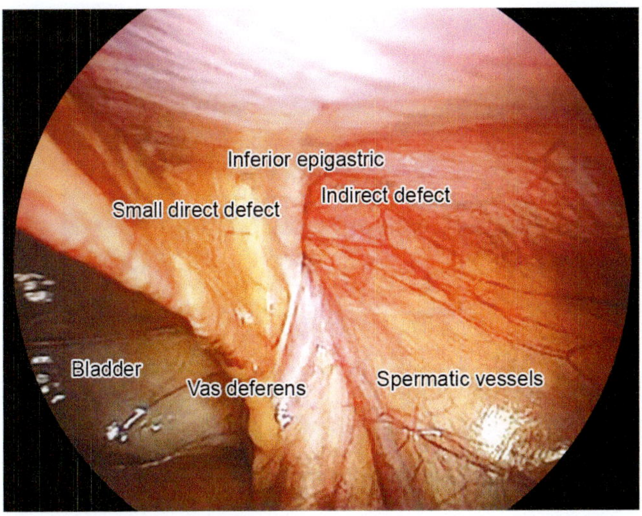

Fig. 9: Inguinal anatomy with the peritoneum intact.

Inferior Epigastric Vessels

The inferior epigastric artery is prominently visualized during laparoscopic preperitoneal dissection of groin hernia.

- It forms the lateral border of Hesselbach's triangle.
- It demarcates between direct and indirect inguinal hernias.
- It leads us to iliac vessels and apex of triangle of doom.
- Bleeding due to its injury can occur during dissection.

Medial Umbilical Ligament

The urinary bladder lies medial to the medial umbilical ligament.

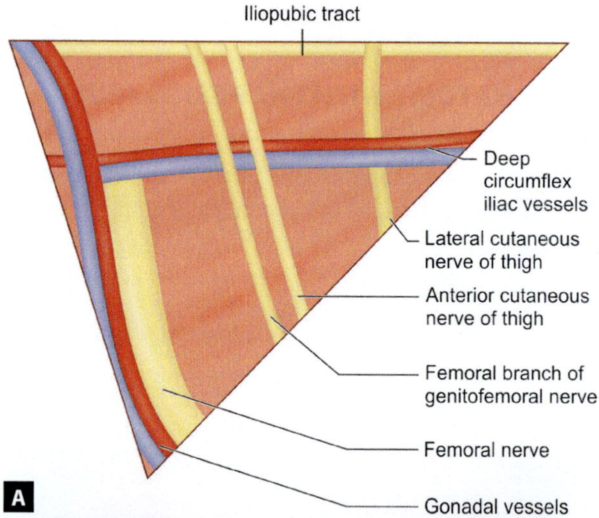

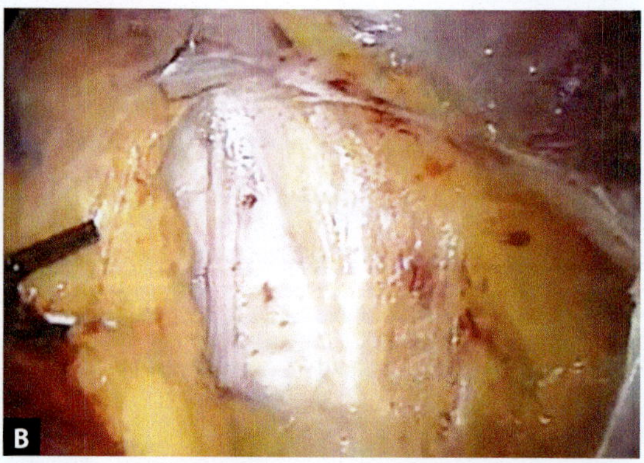

Figs. 10A and B: Triangle of pain.

Spermatic Vessels

Spermatic vessels form the lateral border of the "triangle of doom" and the medial border of the "triangle of pain" **(Figs. 10A and B)**.

Vas Deferens

Vas deferens forms the medial border of the "triangle of doom" **(Figs. 11A and B)** and "quadrangle of disaster."

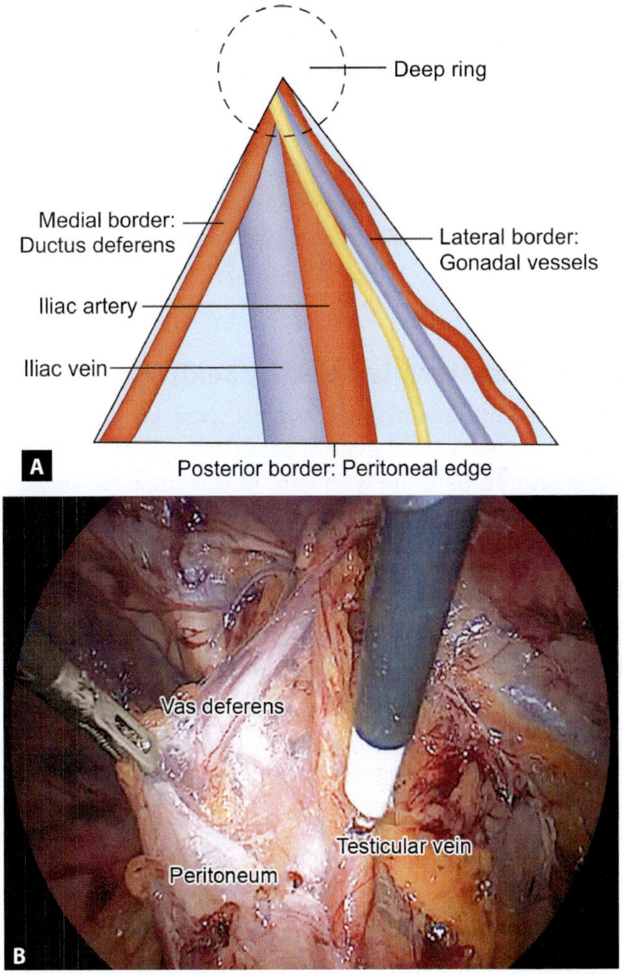

Figs. 11A and B: Triangle of doom.

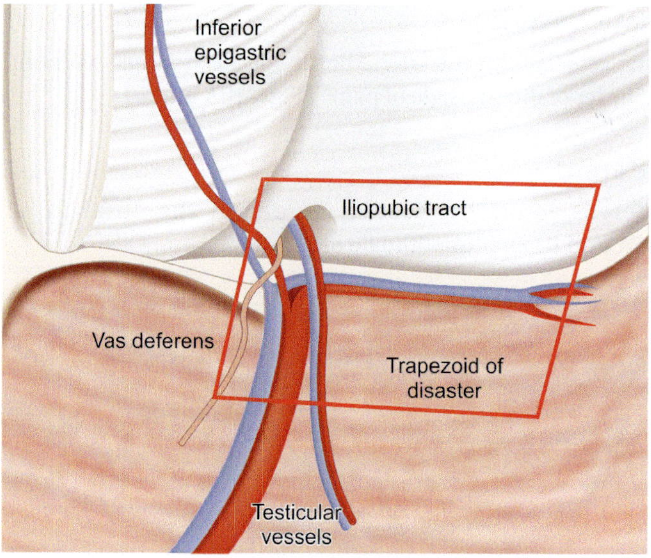

Fig. 12: Trapezoid of disaster.

"Trapezoid of Disaster" (Labeled by Seid) (Fig. 12)

Lying beneath the peritoneum and transversalis fascia are the external iliac artery and vein and nerves—triangle of pain + triangle of doom.

Dissection should be done with care in this area. No tacks should be placed in this area.

INGUINAL ANATOMY—THE PERITONEUM INCISED[8]

After the peritoneum is dissected, six additional structures need to be identified. They are: (1) Pubic crest (lighthouse sign), (2) iliopubic tract, (3) Cooper's ligament, (4) femoral canal, (5) obturator nerve, and (6) internal inguinal/spermatic ring.

1. *Pubic crest:* It helps in getting orientation. Beware of small veins overlying. If they bleed, the entire vision gets spoiled.
2. *Iliopubic tract:* It is a thick, fibrous white tract, which runs from the superior pubic ramus to the anterior superior iliac spine.
   a. The iliopubic tract separates the inguinal region from the femoral canal.
   b. Sutures or tacks should never be placed below the level of the iliopubic tract laterally.

3. *Cooper's ligament:* This ligament is a condensation of the transversalis fascia and periosteum located lateral to the pubic symphysis. It is densely adherent to the pubic ramus and joins the iliopubic tract and lacunar ligaments at their medial insertions. This ligament is used to anchor the mesh in huge direct hernias.

   Mobilizing adipose tissue around Cooper's ligament can injure an aberrant obturator artery, which might course over it. Injury to this vessel results in distressing bleeding. This unfortunate morbidity has resulted in the naming of this vessel as "corona mortis" (crown of death).
4. *Femoral canal:* It denotes the potential site of origin of a femoral hernia. The canal lies posterior to the iliopubic tract.
5. *Obturator nerve:* It courses in the lateral pelvic wall. Mesh placement should extend up to that region. It helps to take care of obturator hernias, especially in elderly.
6. *Internal inguinal ring:* It denotes the site of origin of an indirect inguinal hernia. The most reliable indicator of the internal ring is the junction of the testicular vessels and the spermatic cord in a male and entry of round ligament in a female.

REFERENCES

1. Marks SC Jr, Gilroy AM, Page DW. The clinical anatomy of laparoscopic inguinal hernia repair. Singapore Med J. 1996;37:519-21.
2. Spaw AT, Ennis BW, Spaw LP. Laparoscopic hernia repair: The anatomic basis. J Laparoendoscopic Surg. 1991;1:269-77.
3. Quinn TH, Annibali R, Dalley 2nd AF, Fitzgibbons Jr RJ. Dissection of the anterior abdominal wall and the deep inguinal region from a laparoscopic perspective. Clin Anat. 1995;8:245-51.
4. Rosser J. The anatomical basis for laparoscopic hernia repair revisited. Surg Laparosc Endosc. 1994;4:36-44.
5. Totté E, Van Hee R, Kox G, Hendrickx L, van Zwieten KJ. Surgical anatomy of the inguinal region: Implications during inguinal laparoscopic herniorrhaphy. Eur Surg Res. 2005;37:185-90.
6. Darmanis S, Lewis A, Mansoor A, Bircher M. Corona mortis: An anatomical study with clinical implications in approaches to the pelvis and acetabulum. Clin Anat. 2007;20(4):433-9.
7. Bendavid R. The space of Bogros and the deep inguinal venous circulation. Surg Gynecol Obstet. 1992;174:355-8.
8. Rosenberger RJ, Loeweneck H, Meyer G. The cutaneous nerves encountered during laparoscopic repair of inguinal hernia: New anatomical findings for the surgeon. Surg Endosc. 2000;14:731-5.
9. Annibali R, Quinn TH, Fitzgibbons RJ Jr. Anatomy of the inguinal region from the laparoscopic perspective: Critical areas for laparoscopic hernia repair. In:

Bendavid R (Ed). Prostheses and Abdominal Wall Hernias. Austin, TX: Landes Publishing; 1994, p. 82.

10. Annibali R, Quinn TH, Fitzgibbons RJ Jr. Avoiding nerve injury during laparoscopic hernia repair: Critical areas for staple placement. In: Arregui ME, Nagan RF (Eds). Inguinal Hernia: Advances or Controversies? Oxford: Radcliffe Medical Press; 1994. p. 41.
11. Bittner R, Leibl BJ, Jäger C, Kraft B, Ulrich M, Schwarz J. TAPP—Stuttgart technique and result of a large single center series. J Minim Access Surg. 2006;2(3):155-9.

Chapter 5

PK Band and Other Condensations of Transversalis Fascia

INTRODUCTION

The anatomy of transversalis fascia seen through the laparoscope is unfamiliar to surgeons. It is the main reason why laparoscopic hernia repair is difficult and not preferred by most surgeons. Accurate anatomical knowledge of the preperitoneal area is highly necessary for proper totally extraperitoneal (TEP) repair or transabdominal preperitoneal (TAPP) repair.

The credit of first describing the transversalis fascia and naming it goes to Sir Ashley Cooper.[1] Brause defined it as the entire connective tissue between the transversus abdominis muscle and the peritoneum.[2] There is a preperitoneal fascia separate from the transversalis fascia. This preperitoneal fascia is a thin fascia that covers the preperitoneal fat. It was first described by Anson in 1960.

The transversalis fascia and the preperitoneal fascia are separated by a thin avascular plane, and this space is known as the preperitoneal space. No neurovascular structures cross this space as both are of different embryonic origin. Whether the transversalis fascia proper is bilaminar or unilaminar is still debated. The current concept is that it is unilaminar, with varying amounts of fat on the outer side. Dr Ansari says it to be of three types:[2]

1. A unilaminar membrane with fatty tissue on the outside
2. A unilaminar membrane without fatty tissue on the outside
3. Thinned out and flimsy.

Thus, from outside to inside, the various layers of preperitoneal connective tissue are:

- Fatty transversalis fascia
- Fibrous transversalis fascia
- Preperitoneal space
- Fibrous preperitoneal fascia
- Preperitoneal fat.

Transversalis fascia is not a uniform structure throughout. In the upper abdomen, it is not well defined. It becomes prominent below the arcuate line. Lower down, it attaches to the pubic bone, iliopubic tract and iliopectineal ligament, anterior-superior iliac spine, and iliac crest. It continues downward as the endopelvic fascia in the true pelvis and posteriorly over the iliopsoas muscle as fascia iliaca.

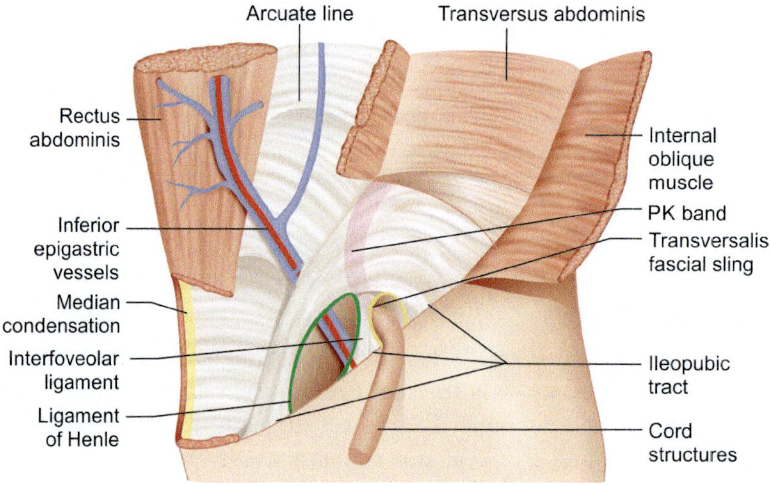

Fig. 1: Transversalis fascia with its condensations.

The transversalis fascia has thickenings at certain specific places, called condensations **(Fig. 1)**. Nyhus, in 1971, gave a detailed description of the "transversalis fascia analogues"[3] in certain areas such as Henle's ligament, interfoveolar ligament with sling and crura, and iliopubic tract. These can be used to close the hernial defect in an open posterior approach. A few other structures that are not a part of the transversalis fascia but could be used to cover the hernial defect were also listed, such as femoral sheath, conjoint tendon, iliopectineal ligament, and triangular ligament.

The retrorectus space is bounded by the rectus muscle in front and by the transversalis fascia behind. Below, it is bounded by the pubic bone and above, it extends into the rectus sheath. The contents of this space are inferior epigastric vessels.

The condensations we encounter during laparoscopic surgery are as follows:

- *PK band:*[4] When we dissect lateral to the inferior epigastric vessels, we see a condensation extending from the lateral border of the arcuate line to the apex of the triangle of doom—the PK (Padmakumar) band. It separates the retromuscular space into medial and lateral compartments. It should be cut with an energy device to open up the lateral space, the space of Bogros. In TAPP repair, we directly access this preperitoneal band by dividing the peritoneum **(Figs. 2A and B)**. The PK band is then split from top to bottom. In TEP repair, the PK band is taken below upward because it is thinner at the lower edge **(Fig. 3)**. At its lowest point, it thickens again to form the "interfoveolar ligament." Histopathology showed a hyalinized fibrous tissue extending from the peritoneum to the muscle without having a fatty layer. Dissection of the peritoneum can easily be done by

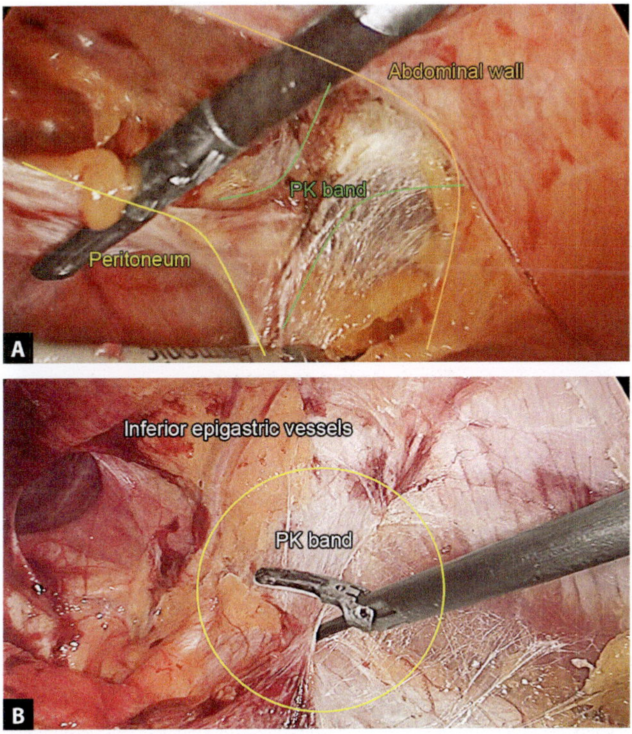

Figs. 2A and B: PK band in transabdominal preperitoneal (TAPP) repair.

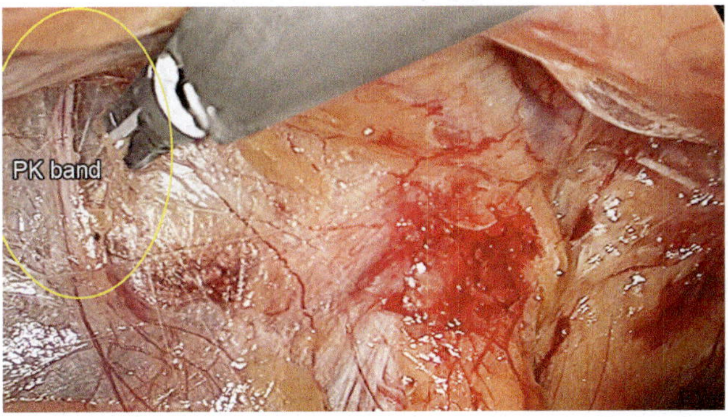

Fig. 3: PK band in totally extraperitoneal (TEP) repair.

dividing the PK band and the remaining areolar tissue can be swiped down with an instrument.

- *Median condensation:* During TEP repair, we see a median condensation while dissecting with the scope from one side of the midline to

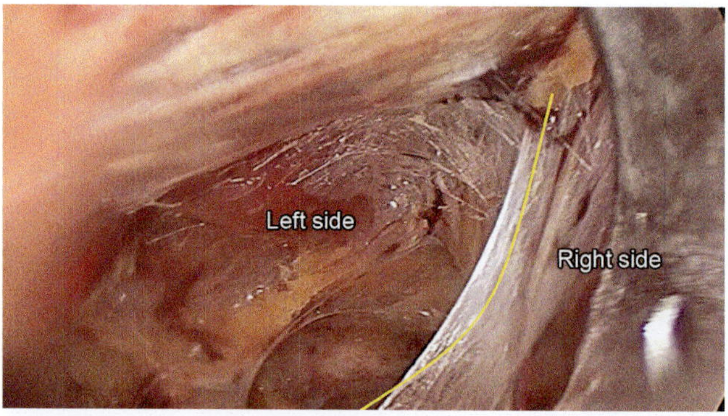

Fig. 4: Median condensation.

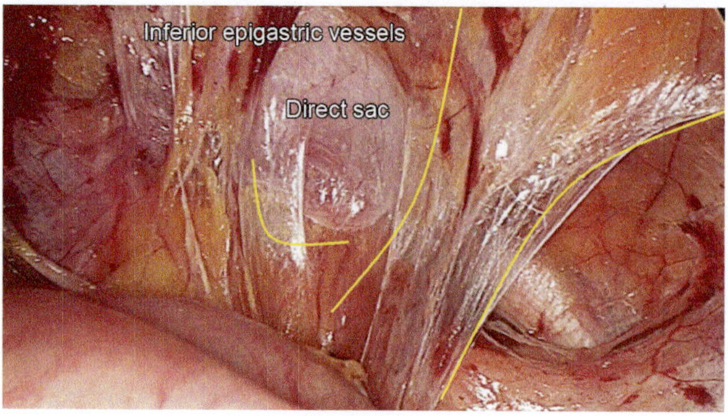

Fig. 5: Ligament of Henle.

the other **(Fig. 4)**. This condensation of the transversalis fascia in the midline extends from the arcuate line to the pubic symphysis. Unlike the PK band, this lies between the linea alba and the transversalis fascia. So, it is not recognized during TAPP repair. We divide the peritoneum to reach the plane between the transversalis fascia and the preperitoneal fascia. Condensation is not visible on that plane.

- *Ligament of Henle:*[1] When a large, long-standing direct hernia is dissected, the transversalis fascia surrounding the hernial sac is found to be thickened. A condensation arises from the lateral border of the rectus muscle, where the conjoint tendon crosses it to form Cooper's ligament; this is Henle's ligament **(Fig. 5)**. When dissecting the sac from the pseudosac, this condensation needs division with an energy device. The urinary bladder needs to be identified and protected because it can be a slider in this ligament.
- *Lateral shelf:* When we swipe the peritoneum over the psoas muscle on the lateral side, the attachment of the transversalis fascia and the fascia

iliaca to the iliopubic tract can be identified. It appears something like a shelf with a fossa anterior to the transversalis fascia and another fossa behind it (the space of Bogros). Once the lateral shelf is divided, the peritoneum is separated, and the femoral branch of the genitofemoral nerve and lateral cutaneous nerve of thigh become visible over the psoas muscle.

- *Transversalis fascial sling:* In males, when the peritoneum is separated from vas deferens and testicular vein, we can identify a sling-like structure that surrounds these two structures **(Figs. 6 and 7)**. It has two crura, above and below the deep ring. This is condensation of preperitoneal fascia around the cord structures. The sling is divided with an energy device and the peritoneum is easily separated from these structures. This is particularly useful in two-port TEP repair, where we have no liberty to use two instruments to dissect the peritoneum.
- *Iliopubic tract:* It is the transversalis fascia that is thickened beneath the inguinal ligament **(Figs. 8A and B)**. This is the structure that we

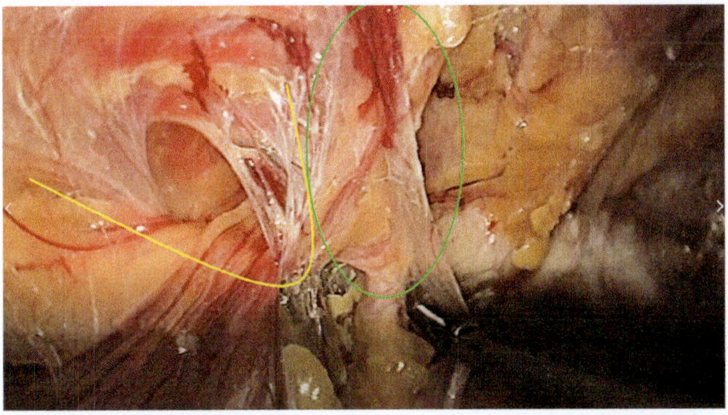

Fig. 6: Transversalis fascial sling (yellow) and interfoveolar ligament (green).

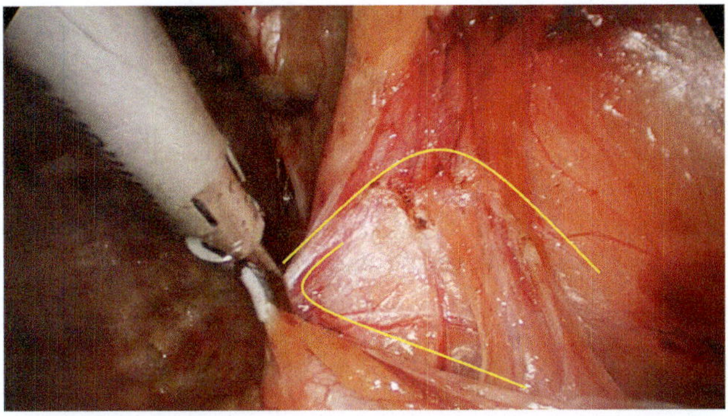

Fig. 7: Transversalis fascial sling (yellow).

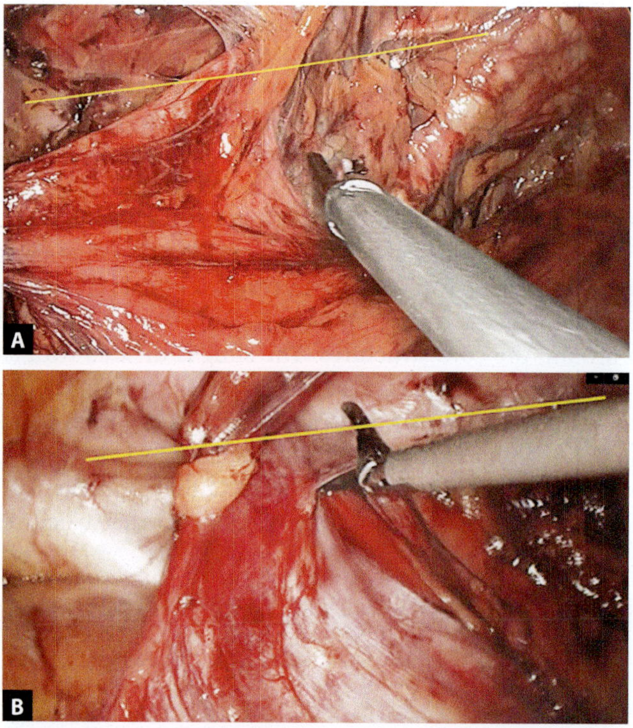

Figs. 8A and B: Iliopubic tract.

usually wrongly call the inguinal ligament during laparoscopy. During laparoscopy, the inguinal ligament is not in view, as it forms the inferior wall of the inguinal canal, and we do not dissect into the inguinal canal.

REFERENCES

1. Memon MA, Quinn TH, Cahill DR. Transversalis fascia: historical aspects and its place in contemporary inguinal herniorrhaphy. J Laparoendosc Adv Surg Tech A. 1999;9(3):267-72. doi: 10.1089/lap.1999.9.267. PMID: 10414544.
2. Ansari MM. Transversalis Fascia and Preperitoneal Fascia: A Laparoscopic Study of Live Surgical Anatomy during TEPP Hernioplasty—Final Report and Literature Review. Ann Int Med Dent Res. 2017; 3(6):SG19-32.
3. Nyhus LM, Condon RE, Harlans HN. Clinical experience with preperitoneal hernial repair for all types of hernia of the groin. Am J Surg. 1960; 100:234–44.
4. Ramakrishnapillai P, Gupta S, Pai M. et al. "PK band" in laparoscopic hernia repair. Indian J Surg (2020). https://doi.org/10.1007/s12262-020-02088-z.

Chapter 6

Transabdominal Preperitoneal Repair of Inguinal Hernia

PATIENT SELECTION

Difficult Cases

- Indirect hernial sacs are closely applied to the cord structures and are more often complete, making dissection difficult.
- Left-sided hernias are more difficult to dissect than the right-sided ones for a beginner.
- Recurrent hernias and irreducible hernias.
- Obese patients.

Direct or small indirect primary hernias in lean and thin subjects are the best during learning curve.

ANESTHESIA

General anesthesia is used.

SKIN PREPARATION

No studies have been conducted to assess the preparation for hernia surgery, but like other surgical procedures, there is no difference in surgical site infections (SSI) in preparation and no preparation groups. In our center, we prepare the skin of all male patients before surgery.

Chlorhexidine scrub bath is given in the evening, a day prior to surgery, and in the morning of the day of surgery.

CATHETERIZATION OF THE PATIENT

The patient is asked to pass urine just before being shifted to the operation theater. Predisposing factors for an injury are a full bladder or a previous exposure of the retropubic space, particularly after prostate interventions, irradiation, or in case of huge or recurrent hernias.[1] If the patient has any of these factors, Foley's indwelling catheter is placed prior to surgery. It may be removed the next morning.

ANTIBIOTIC PROPHYLAXIS

Hernia repair is considered a clean surgery (infection rate <2%). With age >75 years, obesity, urinary catheter, recurrent hernia, diabetes, immunosuppressant/corticosteroid usage, and malignancy, infection rates rise to 14%.[2] In endoscopic repair, antibiotic prophylaxis does not significantly reduce the number of wound infections—level 2B evidence. In the presence of risk factors for wound infection based on patient factors (recurrence, advanced age, and immunosuppressive conditions) or surgical factors (expected long operating times and use of drains), the use of antibiotic prophylaxis should be considered[1]—grade C recommendation. But in our center, preoperative prophylactic antibiotics are administered (ceftriaxone and sulbactam 1.5 g at induction and Amikacin 750 mg the morning of surgery for all). If the surgery time is more than 3 hours, ceftriaxone and sulbactam is repeated.

After induction of anesthesia, irreducible hernial contents, if any, are reduced if possible before painting and draping are commenced.

The patient lies supine with both arms tucked by the side, to make room for the surgeon and his assistant to stand at the shoulder level. The monitor is positioned at the foot end of the patient. The operating surgeon stands on the side opposite to hernia. The assistant, who holds the camera, stands on the side of hernia or behind the surgeon. The scrub nurse positions herself to the left of the patient, to the left of the surgeon **(Fig. 1)**.

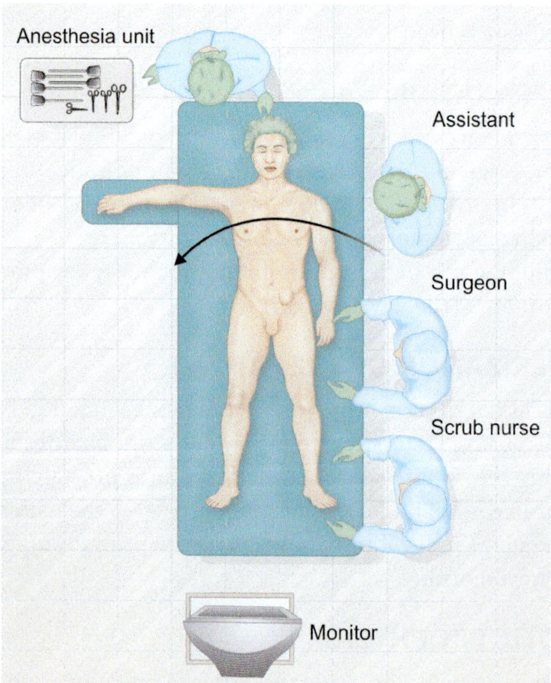

Fig. 1: Cart placement.

PNEUMOPERITONEUM AND PLACEMENT OF PORTS

Open umbilical or Palmer's point entry: Direct open entry with blunt trocar is as safe as Veress needle entry—level 1B evidence.

A vertical umbilical incision is made. The abdominal wall is lifted up and stabilized with one hand and the 10 mm blunt trocar is directed toward the hollow of the pelvis. A 0° telescope attached to the camera is introduced and the entry point inspected. The head end of the table is kept 20–30° low to facilitate movement of the bowel away from the operative field. The groin area is then visualized. Two 5 mm ports are placed as working ports for the right and left hands of the surgeon, one on each side, at the level of umbilicus in the midclavicular line. These ports should be placed under vision to prevent injury to the inferior epigastric vessels (IEV) and the underlying bowel. The telescope is now changed to 30° for better view **(Fig. 2)**.

The hernia defect is inspected, and the type of hernia (direct or indirect) is confirmed by the position of defect in relation to the IEV and cord structures. The spermatic vessels will be seen laterally and the vas deferens medially and they meet at the internal ring (round ligament instead of vas deferens in female). This forms an inverted V. The IEV can be seen coursing upward from this point. A direct hernia is medial to the IEV. An indirect hernia is lateral to the IEV.

All the anatomical landmarks normally seen before peritoneal reflection are identified **(Figs. 3 to 5)**. These include the median umbilical ligament in the midline, the medial umbilical ligaments on each side, and the lateral umbilical ligaments. Contents of the hernial sac, if any, are reduced with the help of atraumatic bowel forceps. In case of irreducible hernias, the bowel

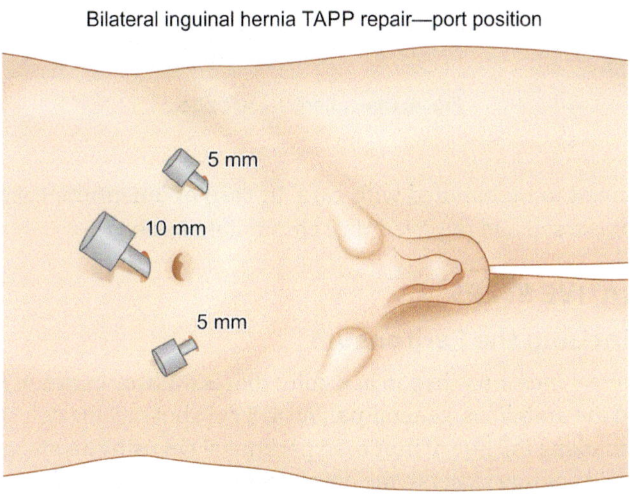

Fig. 2: Port placement. (TAPP: transabdominal preperitoneal)

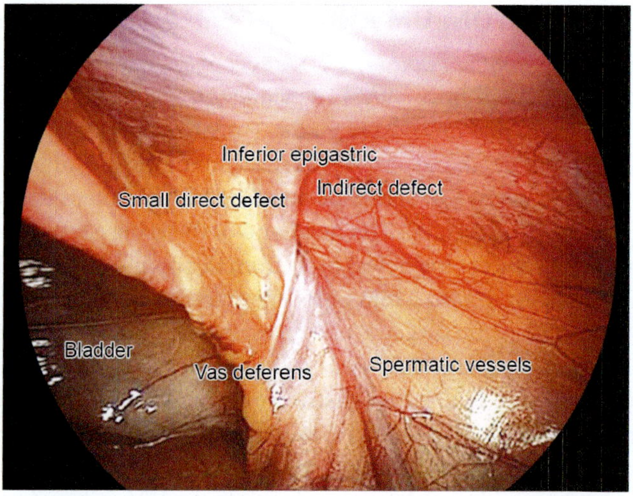

Fig. 3: Anatomical landmarks—right side, indirect defect.

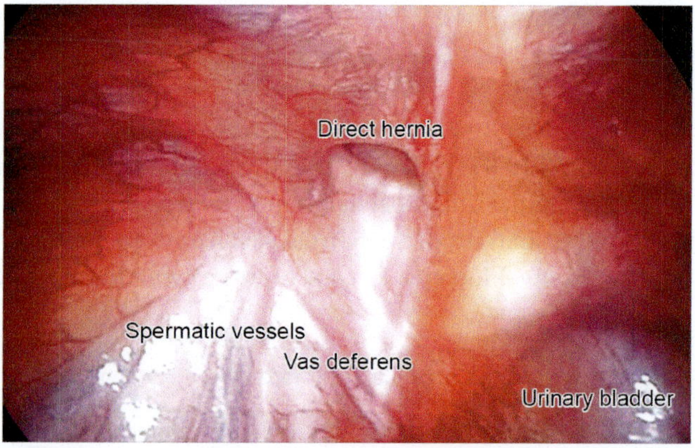

Fig. 4: Direct hernia—left side.

contents need to be handled with care. In case of omentum, they may be reduced or excised and removed via 2 cm scrotal incision.

OPERATIVE STEPS[3]

Step 1: Incising the Peritoneum

The peritoneal incision is begun at a point that is midway between the groin crease and the umbilicus, generally about 4–5 cm above all the defects. It may be worth marking the line of proposed peritoneal cut using an energy source so as to avoid coming closer to the defect later. Incision on the peritoneum is made from medial to lateral, i.e., from the right side to the left on the left side

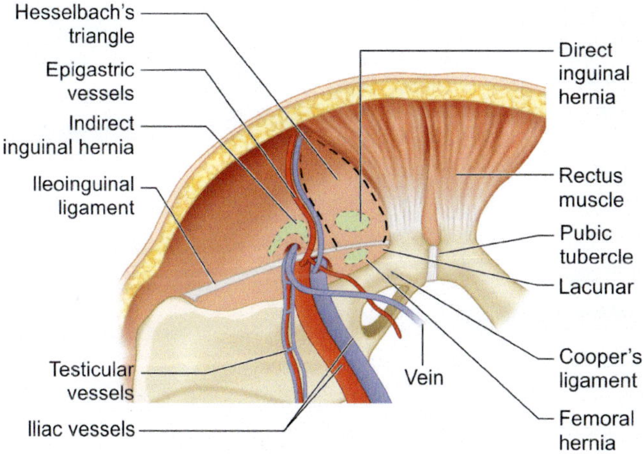

Fig. 5: Anatomical landmarks.

and from the left side to the right on the right side. Scissors, monopolar hook, or harmonic scalpel can be used for the dissection. It extends from the medial umbilical ligament to the paracolic gutter. Extending it medially beyond the medial umbilical ligament may increase the chances of injury to the urinary bladder, particularly if the urinary bladder is not empty, especially if the peritoneal cut is not placed toward the umbilicus **(Fig. 6)**.

Step 2: Raising the Peritoneal Flap

The correct plane of dissection of the peritoneal flap from the transversus muscle is anterior to the preperitoneal fascia through the loose areolar tissue, i.e., in the space of Bogros. The flap is raised by both blunt and sharp dissection. Generally, the plane is avascular, but any small vessel is carefully cauterized before division.

Care should be taken to avoid injury to the IEV while raising the peritoneum medial to the internal ring. These vessels should always be left attached to the muscle and should never be included in the flap. Otherwise, they may come in the way of dissection and may get injured. The plane of dissection is easier on the medial side and blunt dissection is sufficient since the areolar tissue is loose and the peritoneum is not adhered to the rectus muscle **(Fig. 7)**. On the medial side, continued caudal dissection will identify the shiny Cooper's ligament and the pubic bone. Laterally, the peritoneum is slightly adhered to the transversus muscle, and sharp dissection may be required. Take care not to get into the plane of muscles.

In case of local omental or intestinal adhesions to the peritoneum of the groin, it is not recommended to perform adhesiolysis in general, unless it obstructs the view. In sliding hernias or even irreducible hernias, neither adhesiolysis nor reduction is mandatory, but the straightforward

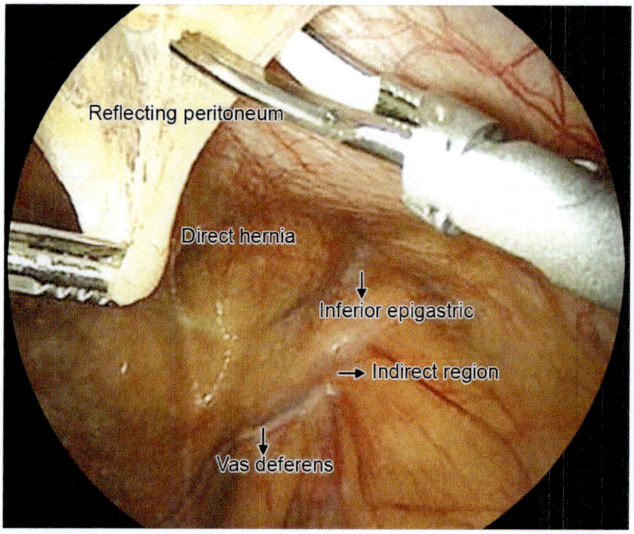

Fig. 6: Incising the peritoneum.

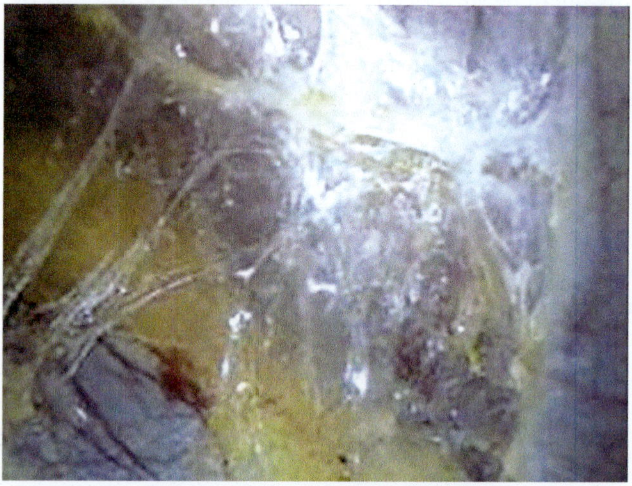

Fig. 7: Areolar plane of dissection.

preperitoneal dissection should be performed. This facilitates the mobilization of hernia content within the sac and helps to avoid intestinal injury.

Step 3: Dissection of Medial Peritoneum and Direct Sac (Fig. 8)

Dissection is continued medially to the pubic symphysis to visualize the cave of Retzius **(Fig. 9)**. The medial dissection should go across the midline to the opposite side, up to opposite IEV, so that the mesh can be placed with a good overlap over the defect. A direct defect is encountered medially above the iliopubic tract. The direct sac can be easily pulled inside along with essentially thinned-out fascia transversalis identified by its glistening appearance and belongs to the parietal wall, i.e., pseudosac. With sharp and blunt dissection, the sac is separated from pseudosac (a push–pull technique). In case of large direct hernias, after reducing the sac, the dome of the pseudosac can be fixed to the rectus muscle over the pubic bone with a few tacks to prevent

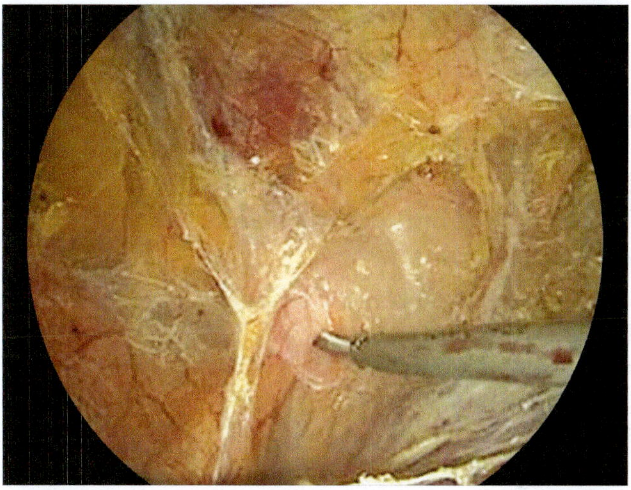

Fig. 8: Dissection of direct sac.

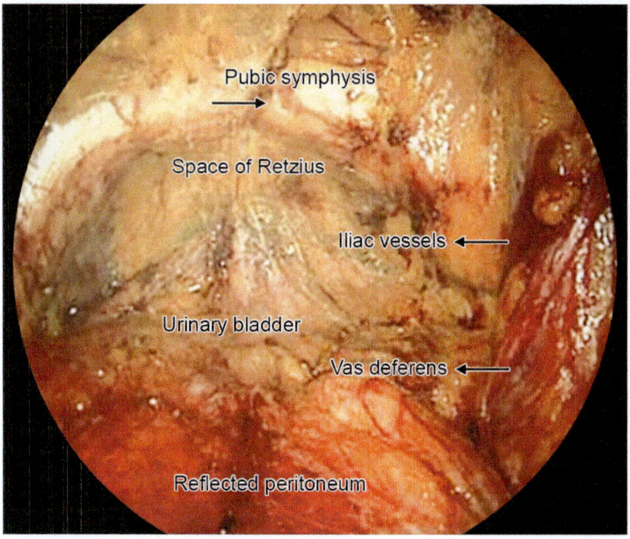

Fig. 9: Space of Retzius.

postoperative seroma formation and also helps to have a base for the mesh—level 2B evidence.[4]

Step 4: Lateral Dissection

After the medial dissection, the flap is raised lateral to the internal ring till the anterior superior iliac spine is reached and it is carried posteriorly over the psoas muscle. Care is taken during this dissection to avoid injury to the nerves overlying the psoas muscle, namely lateral cutaneous nerve of the thigh laterally and the femoral branch of the genitofemoral nerve medially **(Fig. 10)**.

Retroperitoneal area lateral to the cord structures on the left side. The lateral cutaneous nerve of the thigh (1) and the femoral branch of the genitofemoral nerve (2) can be seen coursing on the psoas muscle (3). Both the nerves enter the thigh below the iliopubic tract (4) **(Fig. 10)**.

Step 5: Dissection of Indirect Hernial Sac and Peritoneum over the Cord Structures

Dissection of indirect hernial sac is the most demanding step in laparoscopic inguinal hernia repair and is best done after the medial and lateral dissection has been completed. In long-standing hernias, the sac becomes densely adhered to the cord structures. A grasper is held by the left hand and the sac is pulled medially and the cord structures are dissected away from the sac with the right-handed instrument. A small indirect hernial sac can be easily dissected out into the peritoneal cavity. In case of large/scrotal indirect

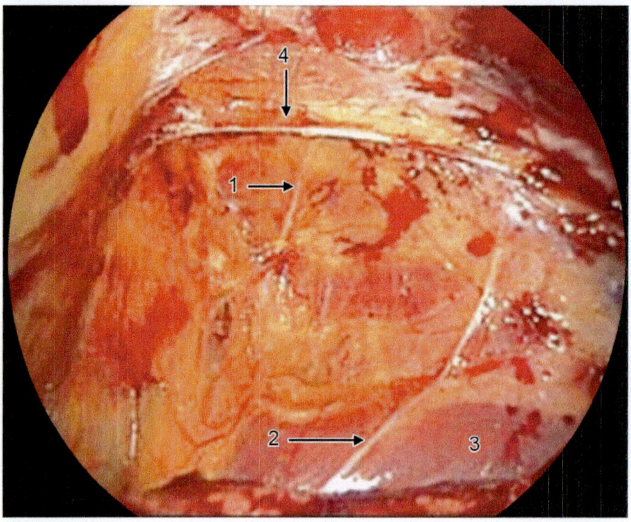

Fig. 10: Triangle of nerves.

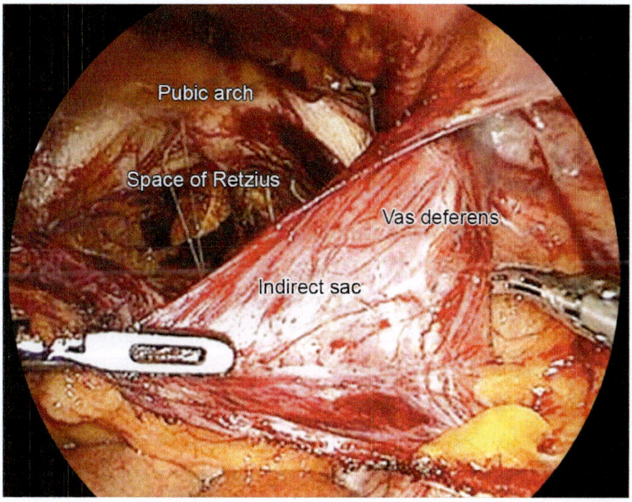

Fig. 11: Dissection of indirect sac.

hernias, complete dissection of the sac may not be advisable as chance of injury to the cord structures is increased and also of postoperative hematoma/ seroma formation. In such a situation, traction is applied on the sac, and it is circumferentially dissected in the "rope-ladder method," so that a window is created between the sac and the cord structures and then the sac may be divided after traction beyond the external ring. Traction will be assisted by external pressure on hernial bulge by the scrub nurse. The distal part is left in situ, but one should ensure that there is no bleeding from the cut end of the distal sac **(Fig. 11)**.

After reducing the sac, the dissection is continued proximally by stripping the peritoneum with both blunt and sharp dissection over the cord structures to expose the vas and gonadal vessels. No dissection should be done deep to the cord structures in the triangle of doom, to avoid injury to the great vessels. Dissection is done till a decent triangle is seen with the vas turning medially and vessels laterally. In doing so, even the flimsiest of the connections between the peritoneum and the retroperitoneal space and spermatic fascia and spermatic cord should be disconnected. A complete anatomical dissection of the whole pelvic floor is necessary for a flat and wrinkle-free placement of the mesh. The extent of dissection reaches medially 1–2 cm beyond the symphysis pubis to the contralateral side, cranially 3–4 cm above the transversalis arch or any direct defect, laterally to anterior superior iliac spine (ASIS), and caudally minimum 4–5 cm below the iliopubic tract at the level of psoas muscle and 2–3 cm below Cooper's ligament at the level of superior arch of the pubic bone.[5] The purpose of "parietalization" is to prevent the mesh (placed over the hernial orifices) from being lifted up by the remaining connective tissue during peritoneal closure; this may especially occur laterally. One should be able to lift the peritoneum without causing movement of the mesh. Any lipoma associated with the gonadal vessels is also dissected and drawn inward.

Step 6: Preparation and Placement of the Mesh

Hemostasis should be ensured before the mesh is placed and any blood/serum is sucked out. If a prominent vein is seen coursing horizontally over Cooper's ligament, it should be cauterized. It may be a source of troublesome bleeding when the mesh is being fixed to Cooper's ligament with a tack. A polypropylene mesh of 15 cm (transverse) × 10 cm (vertical) is used for repair on each side. A larger mesh should be used to cover larger (>5 cm) defects. The mesh is now folded thrice and introduced into the operating field through the 10 mm umbilical port by removing the telescope. The telescope is then reinserted. The mesh is taken to the area of dissection and the middle of it is kept on IEV and then unrolled. The lower medial part of the mesh is positioned against Cooper's ligament. The medial border of the mesh should cross over to the opposite side toward IEV.

Tacks are applied over the medial and upper border of the mesh to anchor it to the underlying muscles, just above the pubic symphysis. Generally, three to four tacks are sufficient, one on the medial border and two on the upper border (one on each side of the IEV). In case of huge hernias, one tack is placed over Cooper's ligament. No tack should be applied on the lower and lateral parts of the mesh below the iliopubic tract to avoid injury to the nerves (triangle of pain). Fixation of the mesh could also be done by using sutures or fibrin glue. In case of bilateral hernia repair, the meshes should overlap each other in the midline and are fixed to each other with a tack so that they function as one mesh **(Fig. 12)**.

Step 7: Reperitonealization

After placement of the mesh, the peritoneal flap is closed over the mesh to prevent bowel and omental adhesions. This can be done with either tacks or sutures. It may be helpful to decrease the intraperitoneal pressure to for better approximation of the peritoneum **(Fig. 13)**.

All carbon dioxide gas is evacuated to empty the abdominal cavity and the scrotum. The ports are removed after lifting the anterior abdominal wall. The sheath at the 10 mm port site is closed with 1-0 polypropylene suture. Skin cuts are closed with subcuticular sutures. A suspensory bandage is used for scrotal support (only if the large sac was dissected). Entrapped air need not be squeezed. Pressure bandage over the inguinal area can be applied to prevent seroma formation.

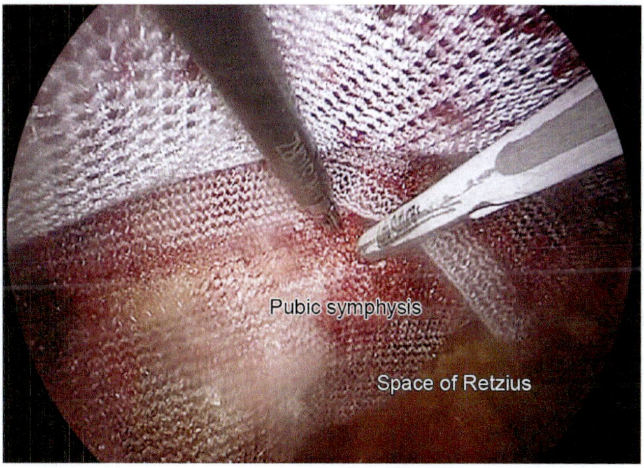

Fig. 12: Mesh fixation.

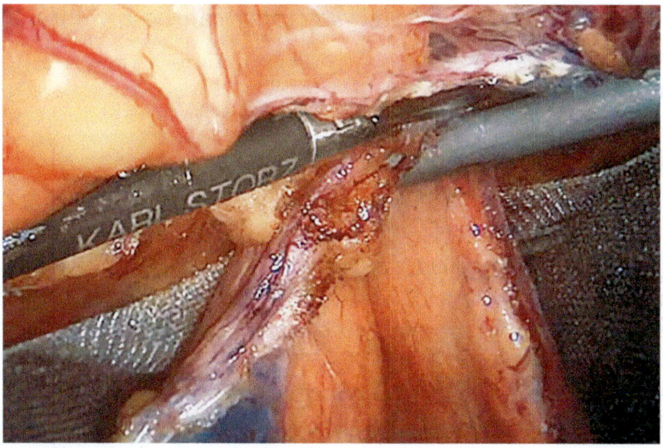

Fig. 13: Reperitonealization.

POSTOPERATIVE CARE

Oral liquids may be started 4 hours after the surgery and soft diet may be started thereafter. Sitting up in the bed and early movements and activity should be encouraged. The patient should walk to the toilet to pass urine. This helps to motivate the patient for early ambulation. Good analgesic coverage with diclofenac sodium, paracetamol, and tramadol hydrochloride, given intravenously (IV), helps in early ambulation and recovery. The patient can be discharged in 24 hours on oral antibiotics and analgesics. The patient is advised to resume full range of normal activities, including driving and sexual activities, in a week or so.

OUTCOME OF TRANSABDOMINAL PREPERITONEAL REPAIR[5]

The morbidity of the procedure is 2.9% and the recurrence rate is 0.7%.

ADVANTAGES OF TRANSABDOMINAL PREPERITONEAL OVER TOTALLY EXTRAPERITONEAL REPAIR[5]

Level 4 and 5 evidence

- Recognition of important landmarks is easier, so it is useful even when the anatomy is altered due to previous surgeries in that area
- Dissection is easier even in cases of bleeding.
- Assessment of opposite hernial defects
- In chronic, huge or irreducible hernias, adhesions between the omentum, intestine, and sac are released.
- No difficulties such as lack of space due to pneumoperitoneum
- Sliding hernia can be recognized immediately and dissection can be performed easily.
- Other surgeries such as cholecystectomy can be combined with this procedure.
- A shorter learning curve.

REFERENCES

1. Simons MP, Aufenacker T, Bay-Nielsen M, Bouillot JL, Campanelli G, Conze J, et al. European Hernia Society guidelines on the treatment of inguinal hernia in adult patients. Hernia. 2009;13(4):343-403.
2. Pessaux P, Lermite E, Blezel E, Msika S, Hay JM, Flamant Y, et al. Predictive risk score for infection after inguinal hernia repair. Am J Surg. 2006,192:165-71.
3. Bittner R, Leibl BJ, Schwarz J. TAPP—Stuttgart technique and result of a large single center series. J Minim Access Surg. 2006;2(3):155-9.
4. Reddy VM, Sutton CD, Bloxham L, Garcea G, Ubhi SS, Robertson GS. Laparoscopic repair of direct inguinal hernia: A new technique that reduces the development of postoperative seroma. Hernia. 2007;11:393-6.
5. Bittner R, Arregui ME, Bisgaard T, Dudai M, Ferzli GS, Fitzgibbons RJ, et al. Guidelines for laparoscopic (TAPP) and endoscopic (TEP) treatment of inguinal Hernia [International Endohernia Society (IEHS)]. Surg Endosc. 2011;25(9):2773-843.

Chapter

7 Totally Extraperitoneal Repair

PATIENT SELECTION

- Tall thin patients
- Good distance between umbilicus and symphysis pubis
- May be done under epidural analgesia in patients unfit for general anesthesia.

PREOPERATIVE PREPARATION AND POSITION OF THE PATIENT

Preoperative preparation and position of the patient are similar to that followed in transabdominal preperitoneal (TAPP) repair **(Fig. 1)**:

- The patient lies supine with both arms tucked by the side to make room for the surgeon and his assistant to stand at the shoulder level. The monitor is positioned at the foot end of the patient. The operating surgeon stands on the left side, irrespective of the side of hernia. The

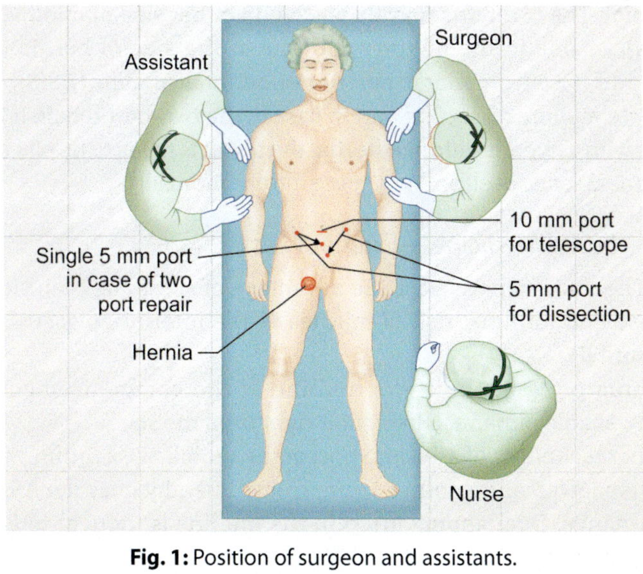

Fig. 1: Position of surgeon and assistants.

assistant, who holds the camera, stands on the right of the surgeon or the patient. The scrub nurse positions herself to the left of the patient, standing to the left of the surgeon.

SURGICAL TECHNIQUE

Step 1: Extraperitoneal Access

A 10 mm infraumbilical transverse incision is made. The anterior rectus sheath is exposed, and a transverse incision is then made on the anterior rectus sheath to one side of the midline to avoid inadvertent opening of the posterior sheath and peritoneum. The muscle is retracted laterally from the midline and a blunt 10 mm trocar is inserted, and a space is created between the rectus muscle and the posterior rectus sheath **(Figs. 2A and B)**.

Step 2: Dissection of the Midline Extraperitoneal Space

Dissection of the extraperitoneal space is done with 10-mm 0° telescope and CO_2 insufflation. It may be done with balloon inflation. The camera is introduced through the subumbilical port and preperitoneal space is visualized. The scope is advanced in the midline till it hits a bone which appears very bright, i.e., "lighthouse sign" **(Fig. 3)**. The scope is retracted a few millimeters and then pushed into the pelvis to enter space of Retzius, about 2 cm below the brim of pelvis. The scope is now moved sideways so that the entire midline is now dissected. The other two working ports are placed in the preperitoneal space. The first 5-mm port is placed about 5 cm above the pubic symphysis in the midline and the second 5 mm port is placed in the midline, midway between the two ports (subumbilical and suprapubic). The two ports may be placed on either side of midline (lateral to rectus), or one in the midline and one at the side of hernia [3–4 cm superior and 1–2 cm anterior to anterior-superior iliac spine (ASIS)], or even just a single midline dissecting port in case of the two-port repair. It is better to ensure with a hypodermic needle that the trocar is going to be placed in the preperitoneal space itself and not going intraperitoneally.

Evidence-based Medicine—Extent of Dissection[1]

Level 5: The midline ports have the advantage of accessing both sides with equal ease and minimal risk of injuries to the inferior epigastric vessels **(Fig. 4A and B)**.

All three ports made in the midline at the commencement of the procedure enable bimanual dissection right from the start.

Another technique of a 10-mm port at the umbilicus, a 5-mm port a few centimeters lower, and another 5-mm trocar laterally near the ASIS is the next alternative. Overlapping mesh in the midline is thought to be easier with this technique.

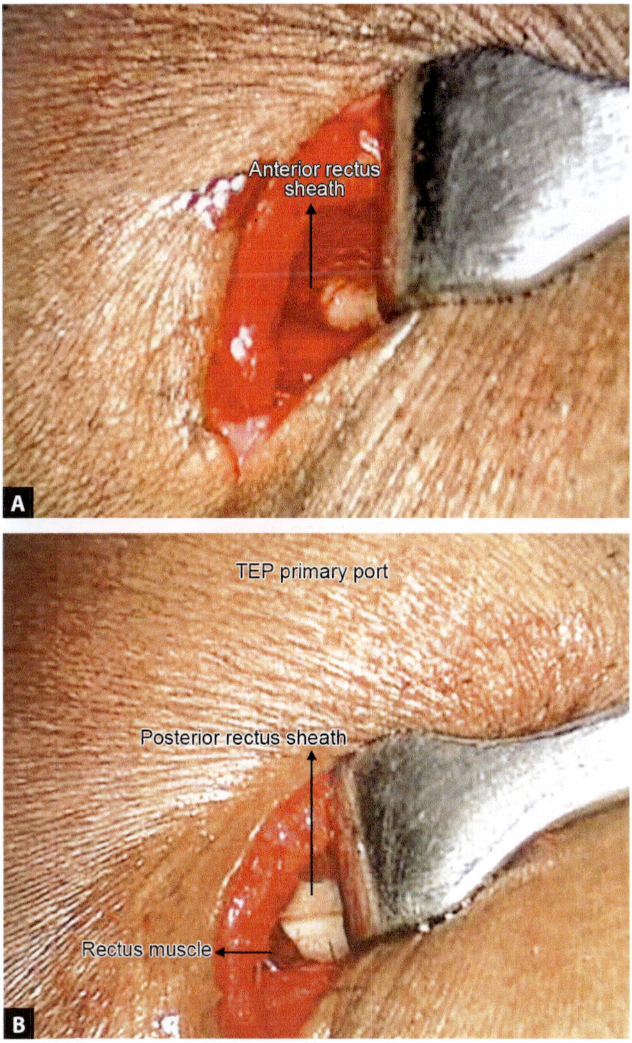

Figs. 2A and B: Primary port for total extraperitoneal (TEP) repair.

Lateral ports, two in number, just lateral to the rectus muscle, used along with a midline camera port is an option.

Step 3: Dissection of the Direct Sac

The surgeon now moves to the side opposite to the side where hernia is present. Dissection is now done using sharp and blunt instruments, i.e., harmonic scalpel, monopolar hook, or monopolar scissors in right hand and nontoothed forceps in the other, dissecting the loose areolar tissue. The dissection is then continued laterally toward the side of the hernia. Dissection

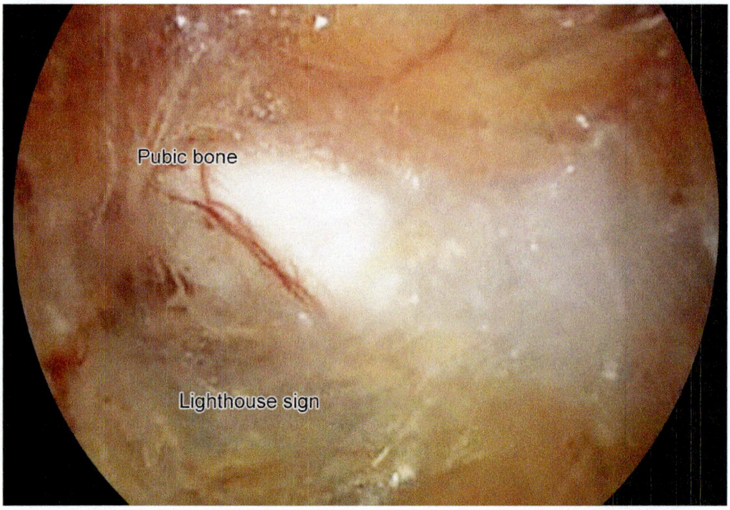

Fig. 3: Lighthouse sign.

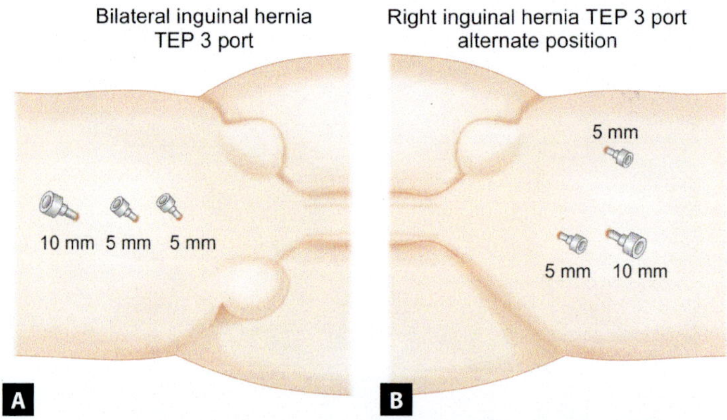

Figs. 4A and B: Port placement. (TEP: totally extraperitoneal)

of direct sac is then done as in TAPP repair. On reduction of the sac, the underlying anatomical landmarks become visible, i.e., Cooper's ligament, iliopubic tract, femoral canal, IEV **(Figs. 5 and 6)**, and the obturator region.

Step 4: Dissection of the Lateral Extraperitoneal Space

Dissection is now continued lateral to the IEV to create adequate space for the placement of mesh. The lateral space contains loose areolar tissue, which is completely divided using sharp and blunt dissection. Lateral to IEV, there is a thick band [(we call it PK band **(Fig. 7)**] which needs to be divided to get into further lateral plane of areolar tissue. The psoas muscle is seen lying on

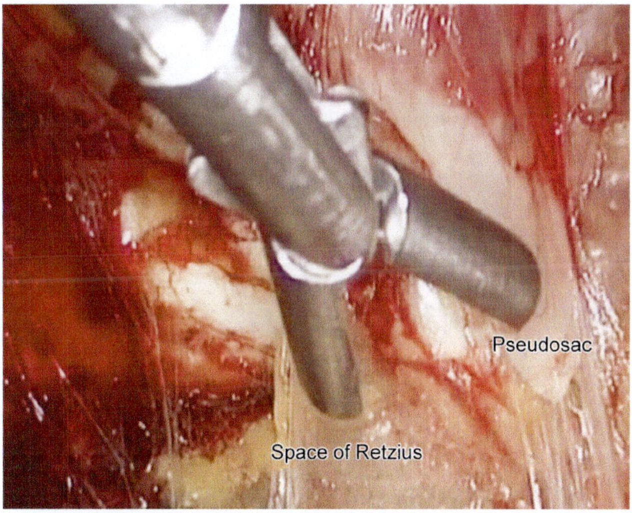

Fig. 5: Dissection of pseudosac.

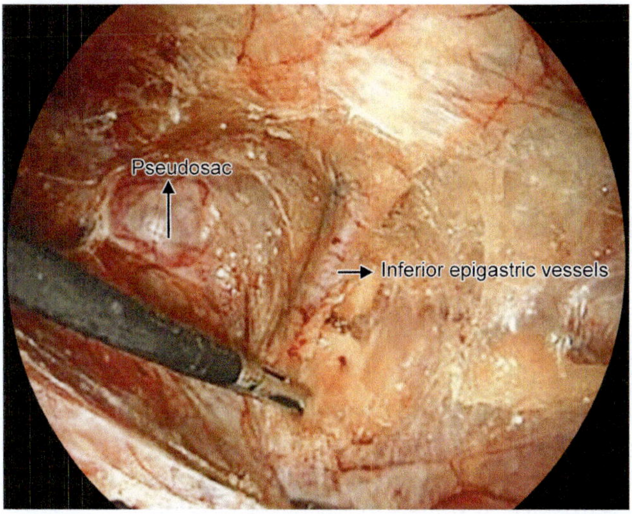

Fig. 6: Inferior epigastric vessels.

the floor where the lateral cutaneous nerve of thigh and genitofemoral nerve can be seen traversing. The ASIS marks the lateral boundary of the dissection. Make sure that you do not skeletonize the nerves.

- The "PK band" is a condensation in the loose areolar tissue between the space of Bogros and the peritoneum.
- For surgeons, the lateral blunt dissection in the preperitoneal plane will definitely be restricted by this band.

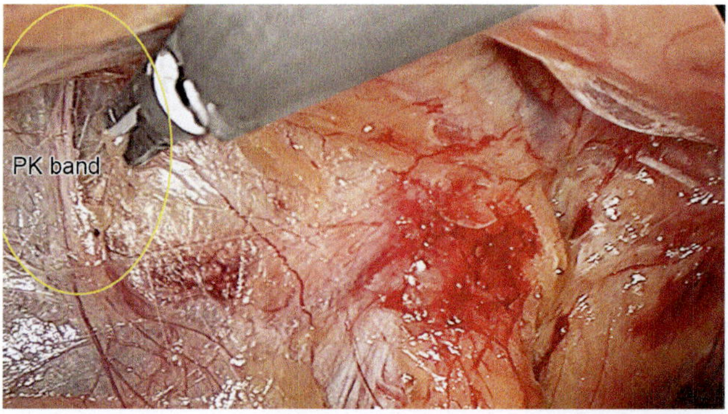

Fig. 7: PK band.

- Forcing the scope laterally will cause tear of the peritoneum at that level.
- The TEP repair space is lost, and the operating surgeon will not be able to complete a good lateral dissection.

Evidence-based Medicine—Extent of Dissection[1]

Level 3: The dissection should extend superiorly up to the subumbilical area, inferiorly to the space of Retzius, inferolaterally to the psoas muscle and Bogros' space until the ASIS is reached, and medially beyond the midline.

The landmarks to be visualized are the pubic bone, Cooper's ligament, inferior epigastric vessels, cord structures, the myopectineal orifice boundaries, and the fascia over the psoas muscle.

Posteriorly, the peritoneum is reflected to the point at which the vas turns medially.

Level 4: Extensive preperitoneal dissection with complete exposure of the myopectineal orifice of Fruchaud is critical to the success of the laparoscopic inguinal hernia repair.

Note: PK band—fondly named by surgical trainees in laparoscopic training course as trainer Dr Padmakumar, who is tough during teaching sessions, insists on division of the band, which yields into easily dissectible areolar tissue plane like an easy surgery following good training.

Step 5: Dissection of the Indirect Sac and the Cord Structures

Dissection of indirect hernial sac is done with a grasper in the left hand pulling the sac medially, and the cord structures are dissected away from the sac with the right-handed instrument, i.e., a Maryland or harmonic scalpel. The sac is dissected from lateral to medial to avoid injury to iliac vessels. In case of large/scrotal indirect hernias, complete dissection of the sac may not be advisable as chances of injury to the cord structures and chances of hematoma formation are increased. In such a situation, the sac is circumferentially dissected so that a window is created between the sac and the cord structures and then the sac may be divided after traction beyond the external ring. The distal part is left in situ. This may lead very rarely to loss of space due to pneumoperitoneum. So, the opposite side dissection should be completed in case of bilateral hernias before you open the sac. The peritoneum will be very loose and hanging now. After reducing the sac, the dissection is continued proximally by stripping the peritoneum with both blunt and sharp dissection over the cord structures to expose the vas and gonadal vessels. Any lipoma associated with the gonadal vessels is also dissected and drawn inward. No dissection should be done deep to the cord structures in the triangle of doom to avoid injury to the great vessels.

Step 6: Placement of Mesh

Gloves are changed before holding the mesh. The mesh is introduced through the 10-mm subumbilical port. The mesh is placed over the space created so that it covers the sites of direct, indirect, femoral, and obturator hernias **(Fig. 8)**. After adequately spreading the mesh, just as in TAPP repair, ensure that the mesh is within the dissected space. The mesh is then secured in place with the help of fixation devices, such as tacks. Preperitoneal space is deflated and reinflated to check whether the mesh gets folded. The port sites are now closed with polypropylene 1-0 and polyglactin 2-0 sutures. Postoperative care is similar to that after TAPP repair.

Evidence-based Medicine—Mesh Placement[1]

Grade C: The mesh should be taken out of its packaging just before introduction under absolutely sterile conditions.

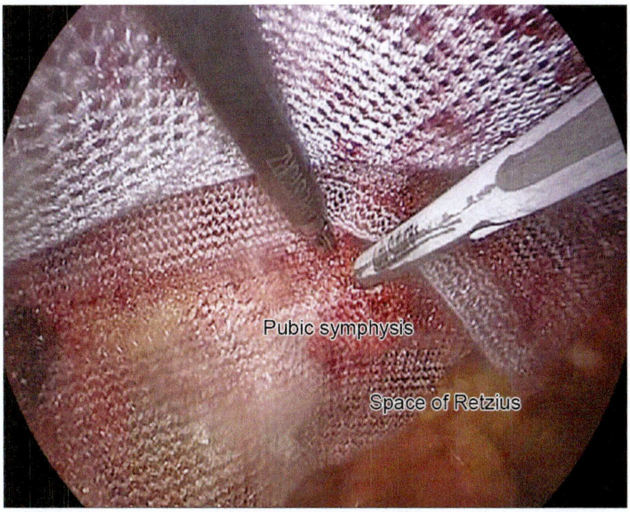

Fig. 8: Mesh placement.

Grade C: The minimum distance between the margins of the prosthesis and that of the hernial opening should be equal to the diameter of the opening in hernias of size 2 cm or larger.

For smaller lesions (<1–2 cm), a minimum mesh overlap of 2 cm is required. For hernias ≥4 cm, the prosthesis should be fixed to prevent recurrence.

Grade D: The mesh should cover without wrinkles all the facial defects in the groin, including Hesselbach's triangle, the indirect ring, the femoral ring, and the obturator ring.

Grade B: Extensive preperitoneal dissection is critical to prevent uprolling of the mesh.

Desufflation of pneumopreperitoneum should be done under vision.

REFERENCE

1. Bittner R, Arregui ME, Bisgaard T, Dudai M, Ferzli GS, Fitzgibbons RJ, et al. Guidelines for laparoscopic (TAPP) and endoscopic (TEP) treatment of inguinal Hernia [International Endohernia Society (IEHS)]. Surg Endosc. 2011;25(9):2773-843.

Chapter 8

Two-port Totally Extraperitoneal Repair

INTRODUCTION

Totally extraperitoneal (TEP) repair is suited for thin, tall patients with reducible direct hernias that are not that large. A 10 mm port is placed in the preperitoneal space in a similar manner. A single 5 mm port is placed in midline. Dissection is as with the usual TEP repair procedure, traction applied with a nontoothed grasper, and pneumoperitoneum applies countertraction. A mesh is placed in the pelvis and then laid to one side using a grasper. With the help of scope and grasper, it is then spread. Tacks are used if required. Patient comfort is very good and with experience one can easily perform bilateral cases also **(Figs. 1 to 6)**.

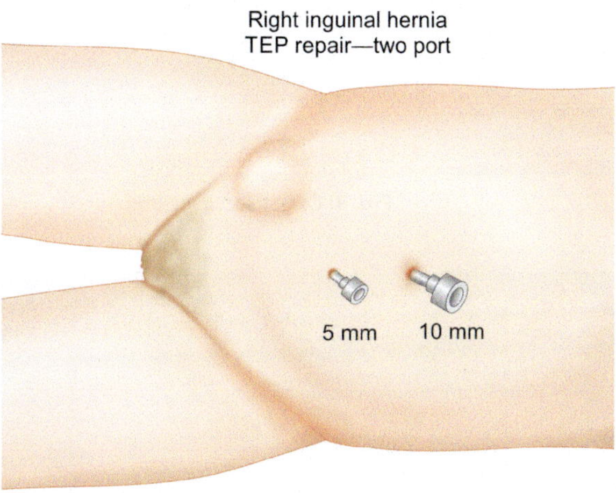

Fig. 1: Port placement in totally extraperitoneal (TEP) repair—two port.

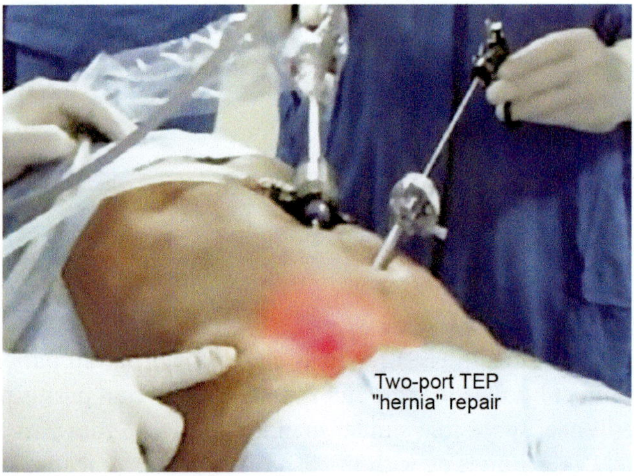

Fig. 2: Port placement. (TEP: totally extraperitoneal)

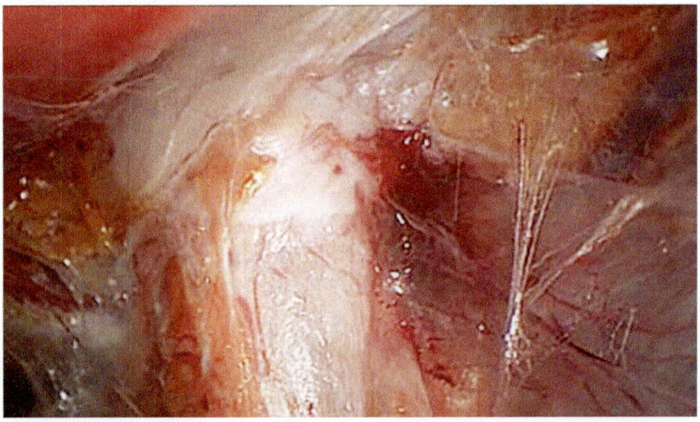

Fig. 3: Direct sac.

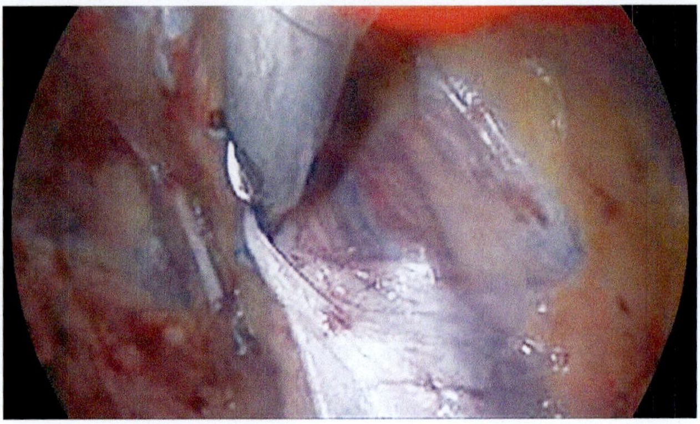

Fig. 4: Dissection of apex of triangle of doom.

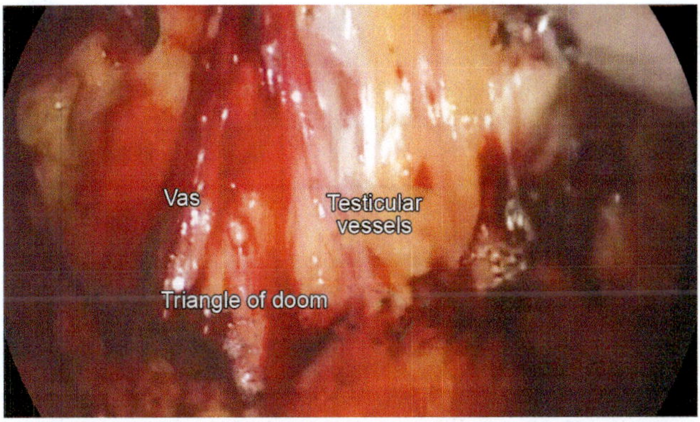

Fig. 5: Dissection of triangle.

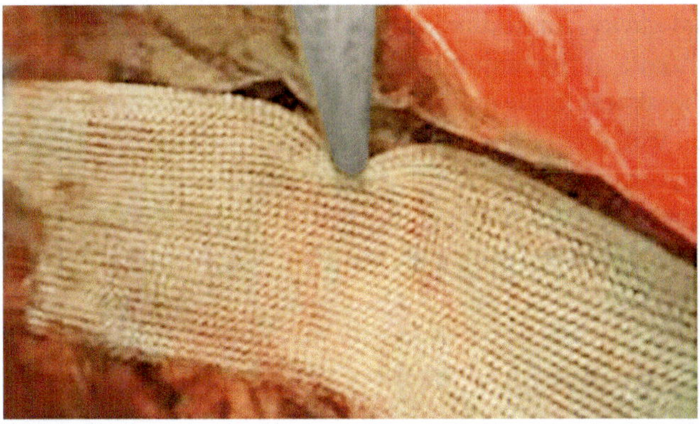

Fig. 6: Mesh placement.

ADVANTAGES

- An assistant surgeon is not required. The surgeon gets better coordination if he himself holds the camera.
- No difference in outcomes when compared with classical TEP repair.
- In difficult cases, the third port may be placed at any stage of dissection.

DISADVANTAGE

Cannot dissect an indirect sac.

Chapter

9 Laparoscopic Ventral Hernia Repair

INTRAPERITONEAL ONLAY MESH

Ventral hernia repair is the second most common type of abdominal hernia operation (25.6% of all hernia repairs).[1] It includes incisional hernia, epigastric hernia, umbilical hernia, lumbar hernia, and spigelian hernia. The abdominal wall is the musculofibrous covering of the contents of the abdominal cavity. An abdominal wall hernia is an abnormal protrusion of the contents of the abdominal cavity or of preperitoneal fat through a defect or weakness in the abdominal wall. A ventral hernia is a hernia of the abdominal wall excluding the inguinal area, the diaphragm, and the pelvic area. Abdominal wall hernias can be of congenital or acquired variety. The latter can occur either spontaneously or after surgery. When they occur after surgery, they are called incisional hernias. 3–20% of laparotomy incisions develop ventral hernia.[2]

When approaching the hernia with the traditional open technique, the fascial defect is ideally repaired with a prosthetic mesh placed in an onlay/subfascial position. However, the appropriate positioning of the mesh usually involves a large incision and a fair amount of dissection, often complicated by the patient's body habitus. The laparoscopic approach to ventral hernia repair offers a minimally invasive technique to repair these hernias.

IPOM and IPOM Plus

When we perform intraperitoneal onlay mesh placement, we call it IPOM. When we close the hernial defect before intraperitoneal mesh placement, the term used will be IPOM plus.

Defect closure ensures:

- Approximation of muscles, thereby regaining abdominal wall strength (abdominal wall reconstruction)
- Prevents seroma
- Prevents mesh cupping into the hernial sac
- Prevents contact of mesh with thinned out subcutaneous fat or skin
- It will give a lattice on which the fibrous tissue can grow and integrate the mesh, giving more strength, thereby reducing recurrence.

Laparoscopic surgery requires much smaller incisions than open surgery; minimal abdominal wall tissue trauma less hematoma and seroma; wound infection was fourfold less likely to occur in patients with laparoscopic repair. Cosmetic benefit varies from case to case (lack of long scar vs. correction of abdominal bulge and a pron). Easier exploration of the whole scar leads to less recurrences, though level 1 evidence is lacking. However, there is a rare, but theoretically higher risk that intra-abdominal organs are more likely to be injured during a laparoscopic procedure. Length of hospital stay after laparoscopic hernia repair was found to be shorter in the majority of trials. Intestinal erosion and fistulization may rarely be seen. Chronic pain and trocar site hernias are to be assessed in long-term trials. As of now, laparoscopic repair can be considered a safe alternative for primary ventral or incisional hernia repair.[3]

Preoperative Preparation

Sequential compression stockings and subcutaneous heparin may be used for prophylaxis against deep venous thrombosis. Intravenous antibiotics (at our center, usually a third-generation cephalosporin and aminoglycoside to cover enteric gram-negative organisms) are administered prophylactically. A preoperative bowel preparation, although practiced by some surgeons, is usually not necessary.

After induction of general anesthesia, the bladder is emptied with a Foley urinary catheter, especially if it is infraumbilical incisional hernia. The stomach is decompressed with an orogastric tube only if necessary. The patient is positioned supine and sterile draping is done.

Operating Room Setup

The surgeon usually stands on the patient's left side, while the assistant is to the right of surgeon. Surgeons may choose to alternate sides later in the procedure to facilitate adequate mesh fixation. The video monitor is stationed at the side opposite to surgeon toward foot end, though may be kept at any place depending on surgeon preference and position of the hernia, in order to facilitate adequate viewing from either side of the table **(Fig. 1)**.

Instrumentation

- One 10–12 mm and two 5 mm trocars
- Traumatic graspers
- Harmonic scalpel or monopolar scissors
- Toothed grasper
- A 5 mm tacker
- Dual mesh of adequate size.

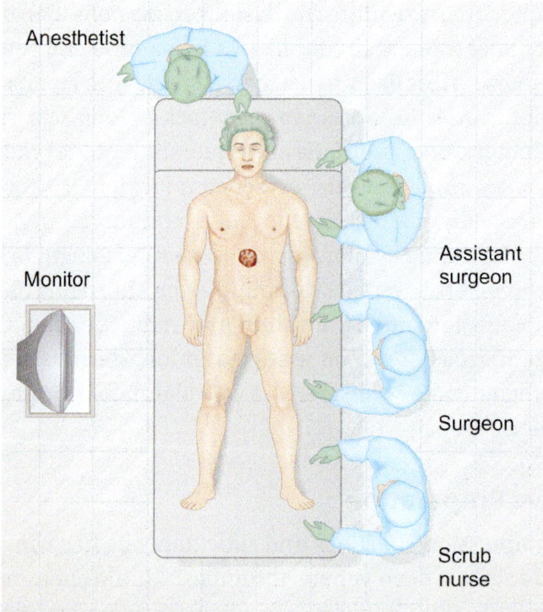

Fig. 1: Operating room setup.

STEPS IN LAPAROSCOPIC VENTRAL HERNIA REPAIR

Access to Abdomen

- Direct entry with safety trocars
- Blunt trocar with open technique
- Optiview trocar in obese
- Veress needle inflation and sharp trocar entry.

Entry should be nicely away from the hernia site. Appropriate port placement varies with each individual operation, depending on the size and position of the hernia as well as the patient's body habitus.

A safety trocar placed in the left lumbar area is good enough for dealing umbilical and nearby hernias. Laparoscope is inserted to assess the size of the fascial defect and extent of adhesions. The two 5 mm ports are then placed under direct vision. These ports must be far enough from the fascial defect to allow adequate manipulation of the laparoscopic instruments and placement of the mesh. This arrangement of ports is called "long" where all the three ports come in an almost straight-longitudinal line with the 5 mm trocars moved slightly medially for triangulation. In case of sternotomy/ cholecystectomy site hernias, surgeon stands in between the legs of the patient with all three trocars coming along a transverse line—"trans." The reverse is done for incisional hernias at Pfannenstiel incision **(Figs. 2A to E)**.[4]

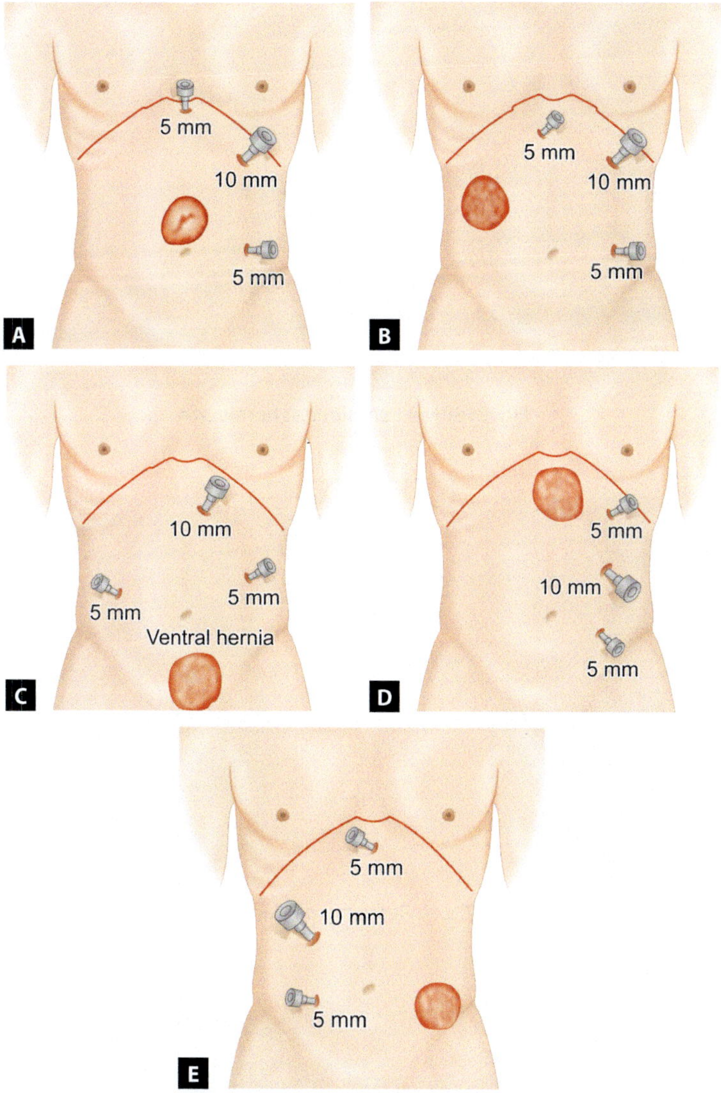

Figs. 2A to E: (A) Port position—umbilical hernia; (B) Port position—right lumbar hernia; (C) Port position—hypogastric hernia; (D) Port position—epigastric hernia; (E) Port position—left lumbar hernia.

Adhesiolysis and Reduction of the Hernia

Using a traction and counter-traction technique, adhesiolysis is performed primarily by sharp dissection. Electrocautery is usually not necessarily due to the relatively avascular nature of these adhesions and should be kept to a minimum to avoid occult or delayed bowel injury **(Figs. 3 to 5)**.

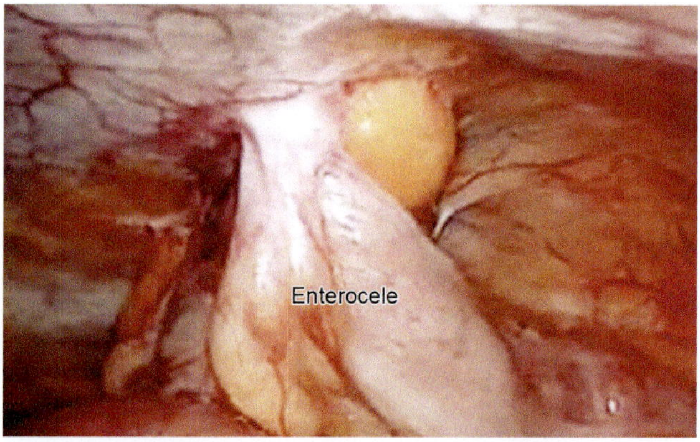

Fig. 3: Bowel adhesions at hernia site.

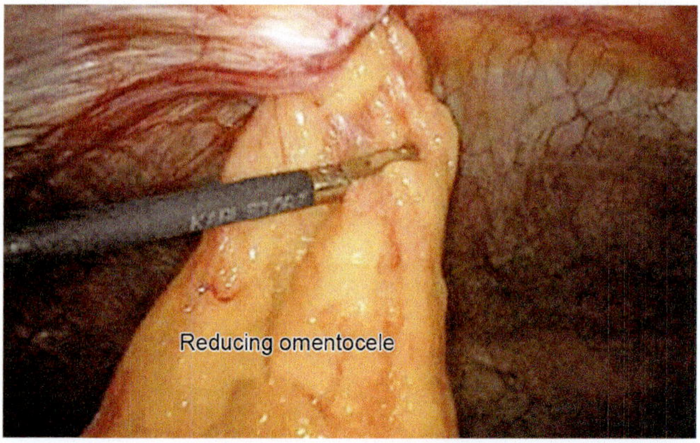

Fig. 4: Reducing contents.

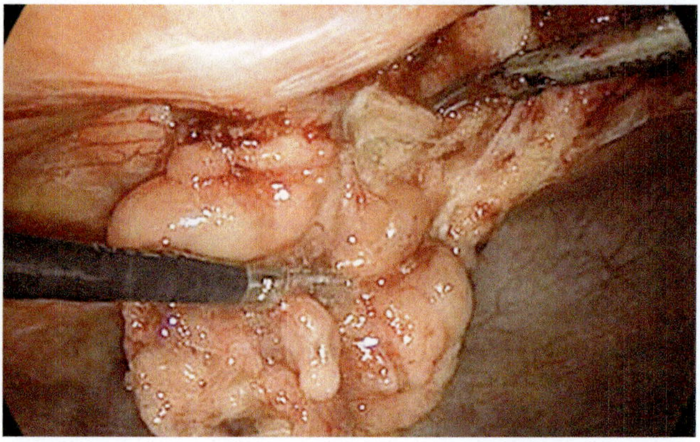

Fig. 5: Reduction of preperitoneal fat.

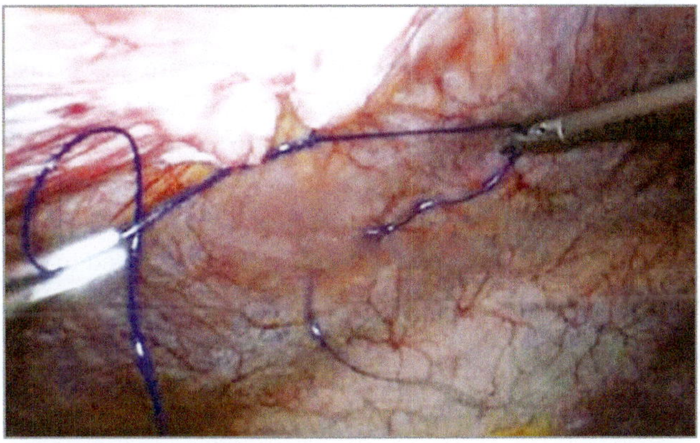

Fig. 6: Suturing the defect.

All adhesions between intestine, omentum, and the abdominal wall should be lysed within a minimum 3 cm circumferential margin from the fascial defect.

It is important to completely expose all fascial defects, as it is not uncommon to have multiple defects resembling a "Swiss cheese" pattern. The circumferential margin is crucial for adequate mesh placement. The peritoneal sac can be left in place unless tenacious adhesions between the bowel and sac necessitate excision of the sac from the fascial edge. Large defect is darned with 1-0 polypropylene to prevent displacement of mesh and its contact with skin **(Fig. 6)**.

Where to Keep the Mesh—Intraperitoneal or Preperitoneal?

Preperitoneal placement of mesh increases the dissection and also the duration of surgery. It gives a covering for the mesh, which can be achieved by keeping an omental cover even. This method is helpful in lumbar as well as very low hernias, where mesh cannot be tacked along one border.

What is the Best way to Measure the Mesh?

There are three options:

1. Extracorporeal with pneumoperitoneum
2. Extracorporeal after desufflation
3. Intracorporeal with pneumoperitoneum[5,6]

With extracorporeal measurement, the diameter of the outer (skin) circle is larger than the inner (peritoneal) circle. This difference is proportional to the size of the patient. It results in overestimation of hernia size and mesh by 1.7–3.1 cm. Size of mesh should be planned in such a way that at least 3–4 cm overlap beyond the defect edge on all sides is present.

Preparing the Mesh

A dual-sided mesh is rolled with the rough side inward and is inserted into the abdomen via a 10 mm port. For larger mesh, either a larger port is used or the port is removed, and mesh is passed through the skin incision in a sterile cover. The mesh is then unfolded and oriented appropriately (smooth side facing the abdominal viscera and rough side oriented toward the abdominal wall) to cover the entire fascial defect. It is placed to allow a 3 cm circumferential overlap from the edges of the fascial defect and the edge of the mesh (15 × 15/15 × 20 cm mesh is the one generally used).

Fixing the Mesh

- Sutures
- Tacks
- Combined
- Glue

Sutures

Sutures are tied extracorporeally, with the knots lying in the subcutaneous tissue, thus providing transabdominal fixation of the mesh at each of these points. For large hernias, additional transfascial sutures can be placed so that there is one suture every 5 cm around the mesh.[7]

Tacks

The mesh is secured by placing 5 mm surgical tacks. The tacks can be absorbable or nonabsorbable. It is placed circumferentially at intervals of 4–5 cm. Another circle surrounds the fascial defect. This forms the "double crown technique."[8] This close interval of tack placement is crucial to prevent the formation of folds in the mesh once pneumoperitoneum is released. These folds could lead to hernia recurrence **(Fig. 7)**.

Alternatively, some surgeons choose to secure the mesh with surgical tacks, along with secondary reinforcement with sutures in each of the four quadrants. Securing with glue is another option.

The trocars are removed under direct vision and pneumoperitoneum is released. Wounds larger than 5 mm should be closed with port closure needle. The skin is closed with 2-0 absorbable subcuticular sutures.

In case of umbilical hernia, a gauze is packed in the umbilicus from skin side to achieve a nice dimple. Application of an abdominal binder is advised in all cases of ventral hernia repairs (laboratory/open) for 6 weeks. In those patients with larger defects, the binder use and rest is continued for another 6 weeks.

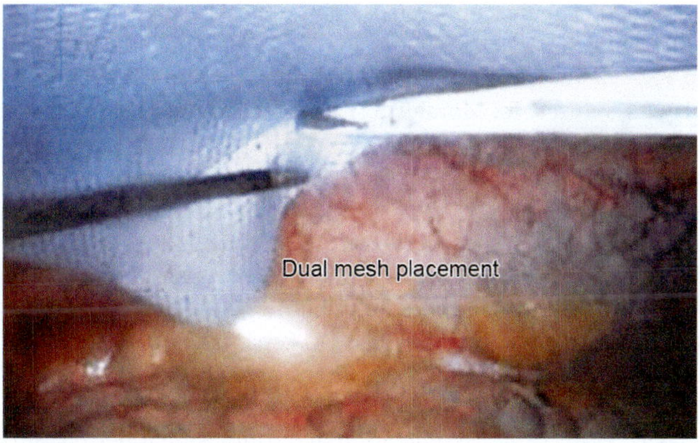

Fig. 7: Mesh placement.

ADVANTAGES[9-11]

- Delineation of multiple small fascial defects
- Coverage of "Swiss cheese" defects
- Avoids dissection through previous operative sites
- Avoids disruption of prior mesh
- No weakening of already weak tissue
- Less pain
- Less wound complications
- Less hospital stay
- Low recurrence rate
- Cosmetically excellent, high chance of retaining umbilicus.

DISADVANTAGE

Learning curve.

REFERENCES

1. Dabbas N, Adams K, Pearson K, Royle G. Frequency of abdominal wall hernias: Is classical teaching out of date? JRSM Short Rep. 2011;2(1):5.
2. Ahmed I, Beckingham IJ. Minimally invasive abdominal wall hernia repair. Recent advances in surgery, 27th edition. CRC Press; 2004. pp. 25-40.
3. Sauerland S, Walgenbach M, Habermalz B, Seiler CM, Miserez M. Laparoscopic versus open surgical techniques for ventral or incisional hernia repair. Cochrane Database Syst Rev. 2011;16(3):CD007781.
4. Miserez M, Penninckx F. Endoscopic totally preperitoneal ventral hernia repair. In: Morales S (Ed). Laparoscopic Ventral Hernia Repair. Paris: Springer; 2003. pp. 283-95.
5. Lauder CI, Strickland A, Maddern GJ. Laparoscopic mesh measurement. Ann R Coll Surg Engl. 2010;92(3):262-3.

6. Jin J, Rosen MJ. Laparoscopic versus open ventral hernia repair. Surg Clin North Am. 2008;88(5):1083-100.
7. Abiad FR, Voeller GR. Results of laparoscopic intraperitoneal ventral hernia repair with sutures. In: Morales S (Ed). Laparoscopic Ventral Hernia Repair. Paris: Springer; 2003. pp. 309-17.
8. Morales-Conde S, Morales-Mendez S. Laparoscopic ventral hernia repair without sutures—double crown technique: In: Morales S (Ed). Laparoscopic Ventral Hernia Repair. Paris: Springer; 2003. pp. 319-33.
9. Heniford BT, Park A, Ramshaw BJ. Laparoscopic repair of ventral hernias: Nine years' experience with 850 consecutive hernias. Ann Surg. 2003;238(3):391-9.
10. Franklin ME Jr, Gonzalez JJ Jr, Glass JL. Laparoscopic ventral and incisional hernia repair: An 11-year experience. Hernia. 2004;8(1):23-7.
11. Carbajo MA, Martp del Olmo JC, Blanco JI, Toledano M, de la Cuesta C, Ferreras C, et al. Laparoscopic approach to incisional hernia. Surg Endosc. 2003;17(1):118-22.

Chapter 10

Extended Totally Extraperitoneal Repair

INTRODUCTION

Extended totally extraperitoneal (eTEP) repair procedure was first advocated by Dr Jorge Daes in 2012 for difficult inguinal hernias.[1] This is useful for large inguinal hernias and also for hernias where umbilicus to pubic symphysis distance is much lesser. When we shift the first trocar to Palmer's point, we get more space for dissection, and we can keep a larger mesh. Later in 2018, Dr Igor Belyansky introduced the same procedure for umbilical hernias and ventral hernias.[1] Later on, it was found that even transverse abdominis muscle release can be performed during eTEP and huge as well as lateral hernias could be repaired.[1] The suprapubic placement of trocars helped to repair epigastric and upper abdominal hernias comfortably. Unlike TEP repair for inguinal hernias, in eTEP, the peritoneum is usually violated, especially at the hernial region. This opening can be used to check for adhesions, and adhesiolysis can be performed. The advantages of eTEP are that the regular polypropylene mesh can be used for ventral hernias and it can be placed extraperitoneally.

ANATOMY OF THE ANTERIOR ABDOMINAL WALL

The anterior abdominal wall is formed of two aponeurotic fibrous tissues—anterior and posterior rectus sheaths.[2] In between these, there is rectus abdominis muscle on either side. Laterally, the anterior abdominal wall is formed by three layers of muscles, namely the external oblique, the internal oblique, and the transversus abdominis. In the midline, anterior and posterior rectus sheaths fuse to form the linea alba. Just lateral to the border of the rectus muscle again these fibrotic aponeurotic tissues merge together to form the linea semilunaris. The linea alba and the linea semilunaris run parallelly. Linea alba extends in the midline from the xiphisternum to the pubic symphysis **(Fig. 1)**. Linea semilunaris extends from the rib cage to the pelvic rim, lateral to the lateral border of the rectus abdominis muscle **(Fig. 1)**. The posterior rectus sheath starts from the xiphisternum and ends approximately one third between umbilicus and pubic symphysis. This lower border of the posterior rectus sheath is known as the arcuate line or the semicircular line of Douglas. Below the arcuate line, the posterior rectus sheath is deficient; instead, transversalis fascia strengthens the abdominal wall.

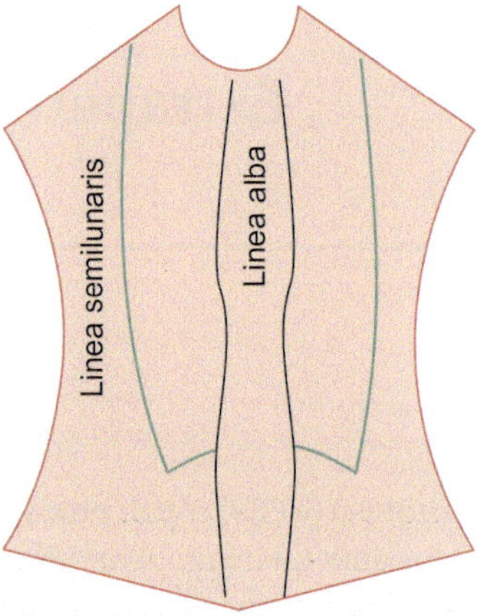

Fig. 1: Extent of linea alba and linea semilunaris.

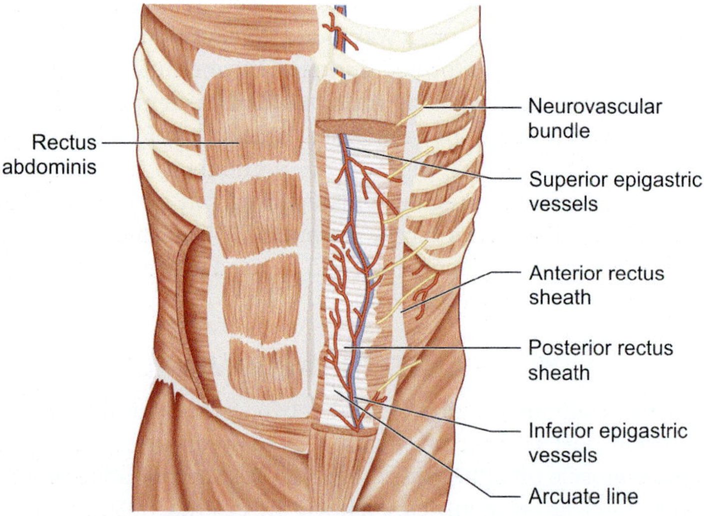

Fig. 2: Anatomy of retrorectus space.

Retrorectus Space[3]

Retrorectus space is a potential space, bounded posteriorly by the posterior rectus sheath and the transversalis fascia and anteriorly by the rectus muscle. The space extends superiorly up to the rib cage and inferiorly to the pelvic brim. Laterally, it extends up to the linea semilunaris. Medially, it ends where anterior and posterior rectus sheaths fuse to form the linea alba. The contents of each retrorectus space are superior and inferior epigastric vessels and five neurovascular structures, which supply the rectus abdominis muscle **(Figs. 2 and 3)**.

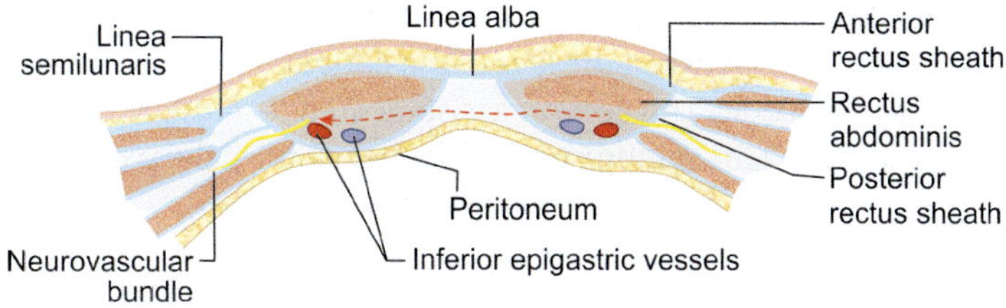

Fig. 3: Cross-sectional view of the anterior abdominal wall showing the line of dissection.

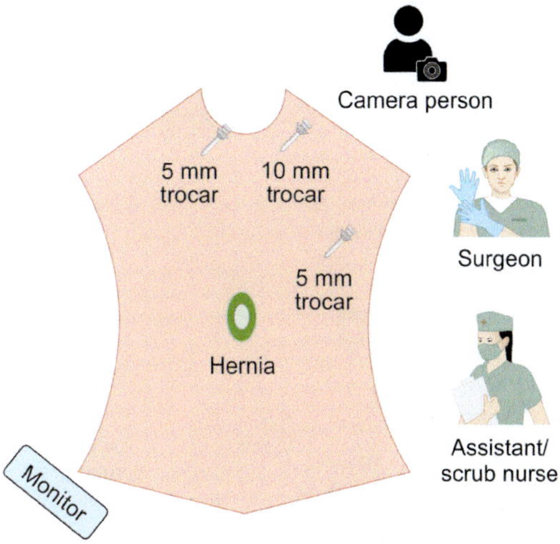

Fig. 4: Position of team and trocars in umbilical or subumbilical hernia.

PREOPERATIVE PREPARATION

Just like intraperitoneal onlay mesh (IPOM),

- Chlorhexidine scrub bath in the evening, a day prior to surgery, and in the morning of the day of surgery
- Prophylactic antibiotics on the day of surgery
- NPO
- The patient is under general anesthesia (GA)
- Ryle's tube, if needed
- Made to pass urine just before being taken to the operation theater (OT), or else catheterize on the table
- Patient is kept supine.

If the hernia is at the level of the umbilicus or below that, the surgeon stands on the left of the patient near the shoulder. A laparoscopic cart is kept at the right side toward the foot of the patient. The assistant stands to the right of the surgeon. The scrub nurse stands to the left **(Fig. 4)**.

If the hernia is in the epigastric region or even just above the umbilicus, the surgeon stands in between the legs of the patient. The assistant stands to the right of the surgeon. The second assistant stands to the left. The cart is kept toward the left of the midline toward the head end of the patient **(Fig. 5)**. Trocar placements also vary in these two approaches.

Marking

After cleaning and draping, the defect is marked. The proposed site of mesh placement is also marked on the anterior abdominal wall with 5 cm overlap. This helps in orienting the mesh inside with a hypodermic needle. This also helps in limiting the dissection to what is sufficient **(Fig. 6)**.

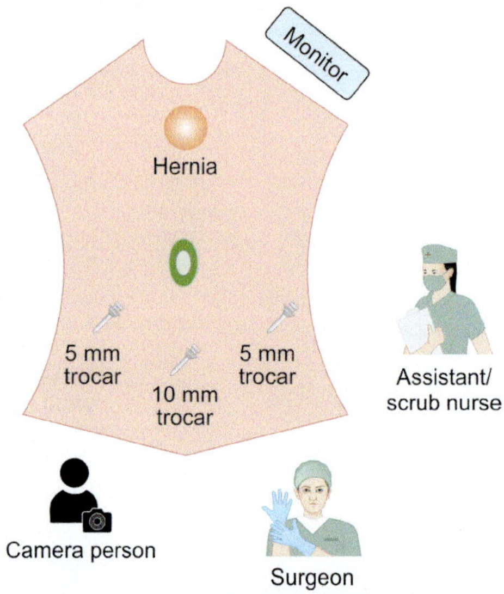

Fig. 5: Position of team and trocars in epigastric hernia.

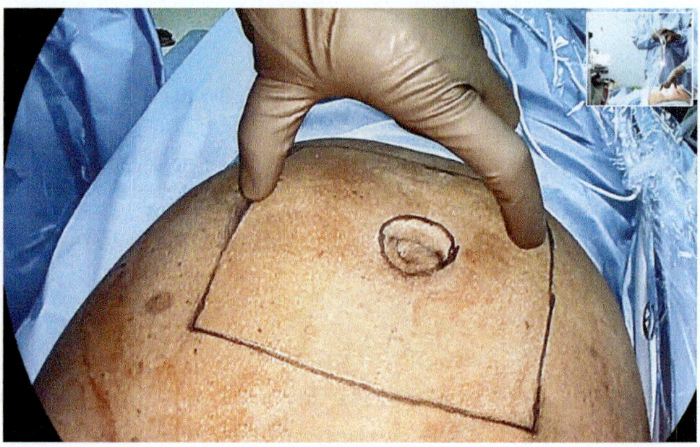

Fig. 6: Marking.

OPERATIVE STEPS

Placement of the First Trocar

A transverse incision is made, sufficient to introduce a 10 mm trocar either in the epigastrium or in the suprapubic region. A 10 mm Optiview trocar is introduced approximately 5 cm to the left of midline in Palmer's point or in the suprapubic region along the midline. Introduction of the trocar should be with a screwing movement, visualizing layer by layer. Once the rectus abdominis muscle is crossed, we should make the trocar parallel to the abdominal wall so that the posterior rectus sheath is not pierced. The trocar is pushed inside between the posterior rectus sheath and the rectus abdominis muscle. Once the sheath is inside the retrorectus space, the obturator is removed and carbon dioxide is inflated.

Creation of Retrorectus Space (Left)

Blunt dissection, using a 10 mm 0° telescope, is continued till the entire left retrorectus space is dissected. The skin marking guides us in limiting our dissection. If we puncture the posterior rectus sheath and enter the peritoneum, we abandon eTEP and proceed with IPOM or TARM repair.

Placement of Second Trocar

Once adequate dissection of the left retrorectus space is done, the second trocar is placed, confirming the position using a hypodermic needle. A 5 mm trocar is introduced laterally into the retrorectus space somewhere at the level of umbilicus or in the suprapubic crease. The trocar is positioned >5 cm away from the first trocar so that there is no crowding of instruments. During the introduction of the trocar, we should be careful not to injure the inferior epigastric vessels **(Fig. 7)**.

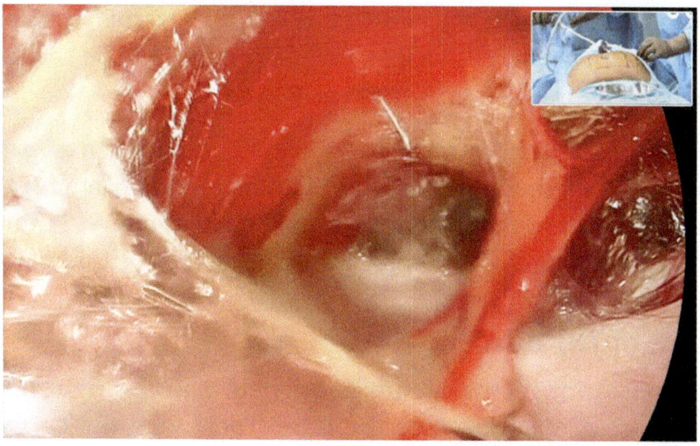

Fig. 7: Placement of secondary trocar.

Dissection with an Ultrasonic Shear

An ultrasonic shear is introduced in the 5 mm trocar and the dissection of the space, which is marked on the left side, is completed. Usually, we do not dissect lateral to the inferior epigastric vessels. If we keep ourselves between both inferior epigastric vessels, even a mesh of size 10 × 15 cm can be comfortably placed. If we want to place a larger mesh 12 × 15 cm, or 15 × 15 cm, we have to dissect the inferior epigastric vessels and go toward the lateral aspect of the retrorectus space. When such dissection is performed, we have to specifically identify neurovascular bundles at multiple levels, entering the rectus muscle and keeping them safe. Once injured, it leads to paralysis of rectus muscle and leads to recurrence of hernia.

Division of the Left Posterior Rectus Sheath

As we approach the medial border of the rectus muscle, a point is reached where we cannot proceed more medially because the anterior and posterior rectus sheaths merge together. One appreciates that the posterior rectus sheath is going medially and deep to the rectus muscle. At that region, divide the posterior rectus sheath just 2 mm away from the border. This division can be performed either in epigastrium, if you are standing on the head end of the patient, or in the lower part at the arcuate ligament, if we are standing between the legs of the patient. Then, the posterior rectus sheath is divided either below upward or above downward.

Crossover and Dissection of the Hernia

Dissect the preperitoneal space and push down the fat and peritoneum. Push anteriorly the linea alba. When the site of umbilicus or the hernia is reached, mostly we open up the peritoneal cavity. The contents of hernia as well as adhesions can be examined and released. Through that opening, we can enter the peritoneal cavity and view the inside. By this time, half of the dissection is over and with its weight, the peritoneum will be hanging down, even if there is pneumoperitoneum **(Figs. 8A to C)**.

Crossover: The junction between the linea alba and the posterior rectus sheath is made out where the criss-cross fibers of the linea alba change to horizontal fibers. The right posterior rectus sheath is entered 2 mm down. A small cut is made on the posterior rectus sheath of the right side.

Placement of Third Trocar

The entire posterior rectus sheath is opened, and the right retrorectus space is dissected. We introduce the third trocar with the guidance of a hypodermic needle to mark its position. A 5 mm trocar is introduced either

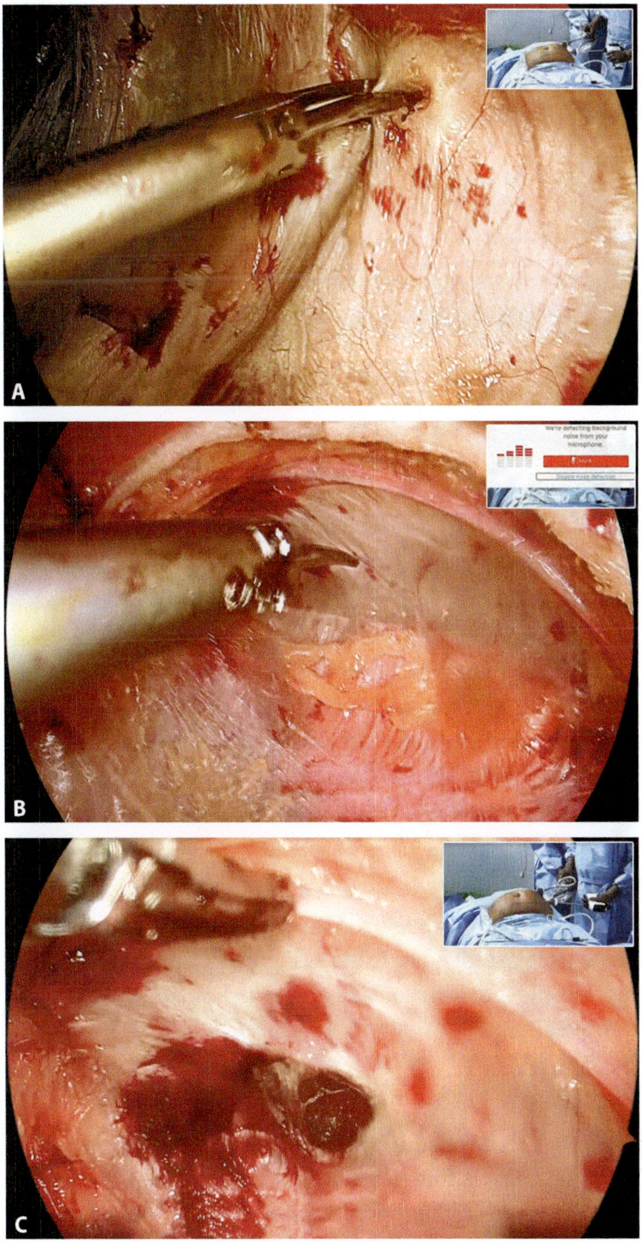

Figs. 8A to C: Crossover.

in the epigastric region or in the suprapubic crease. The dissection should be restricted as per the marking made. The neurovascular bundles along with superior and inferior epigastric vessels are preserved **(Fig. 9)**.

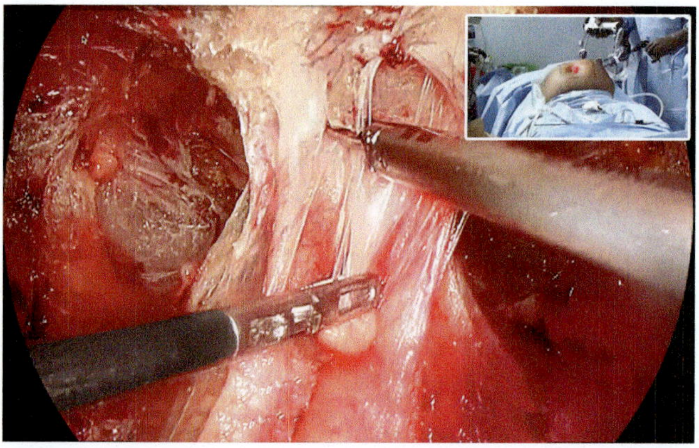

Fig. 9: Dissection of umbilicus.

TRANSVERSUS ABDOMINIS RELEASE

In a lumbar hernia or a large midline hernia where the defect could not be closed, we may need to dissect the lateral space by transversus abdominis muscle release. This can be done either on one side or on both sides. Just below the emerging neurovascular bundles, we can identify the transversus abdominis muscle getting to the posterior rectus sheath. At this level, the muscle is divided from the arcuate line to the rib cage, to reach the preperitoneal space **(Fig. 10)**. The loose areolar tissue in the lateral abdominal space gets opened up so that a very large-sized mesh can be placed.

Suturing of Defects

There are seven types of defects. The reasons for closing them and the material to be used are given in **Table 1, Figures 11 and 12**.

Sutures are placed from either below up or above down as per the surgeon's convenience.

Mesh Placement

The next step in this procedure is the mesh placement. A polypropylene mesh of adequate size is folded and introduced through the 10 mm trocar. The mesh is deployed in the dissected space. If the dissected space is just adequate, there is no need for mesh fixation as the mesh will stay inside the dissected space itself. If the dissection area is more, then we have to fix the mesh using two tacks or stitches. Or else, we have to keep a larger mesh to cover the entire dissected area. The CO_2 is then deflated and inflated again to confirm whether the mesh is placed in the correct position and there is no folding of the mesh **(Fig. 13)**.

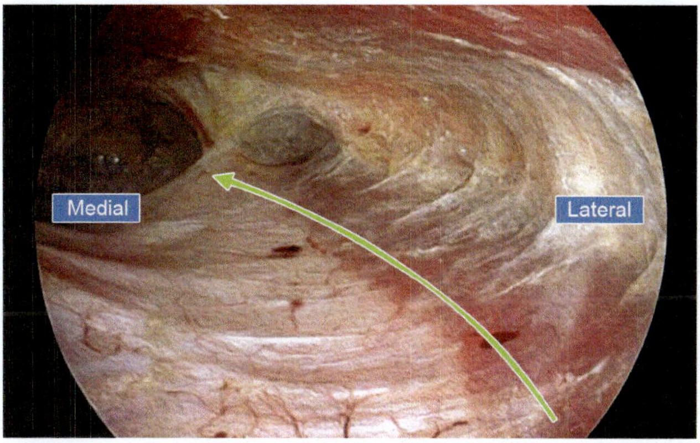

Fig. 10: Line of division of transversus abdominis release (TAR).

TABLE 1: Various defects and the method of suturing.

Defects	*Materials used*	*Tips*	*Absolute/optional*
Hernial defect on the anterior rectus sheath	0 V-Loc PBT 15 cm	• It avoids mesh cupping • Gives a strong tissue on which the mesh can integrate • At umbilicus, dermal bite is taken for cosmesis and obliteration of the space to avoid seroma	Absolute based on the site and size
Buttonholes on the linea alba during dissection	0 V-Loc PBT 15 cm	It avoids mesh cupping	Absolute based on the site and size
Swiss cheese defects	0 V-Loc PBT 15 cm	It avoids mesh cupping	Absolute based on the site and size
Divarication recti	0 V-Loc PBT 45 cm	• For cosmesis • Ridge formation may develop • Abdominoplasty/hybrid may be a better option	Optional
Hernial defect on the posterior rectus sheath	0 V-Loc PBT 15 cm	For peritoneal closure to prevent mesh exposure	Absolute
Peritoneal rents	0 V-Loc PBT 15 cm	For peritoneal closure to prevent mesh exposure	Absolute
Gap between the posterior rectus sheaths and the site of TAR	• 0 V-Loc PBT 45 cm • Stapler	The sheath edges will get adherent with the mesh and strength regained	Optional

(PBT: polybutylene terephthalate; TAR: transversus abdominis release)

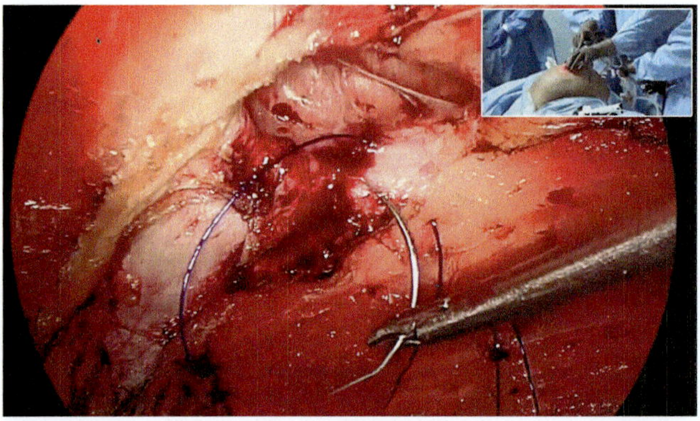

Fig. 11: Closing of umbilical defect.

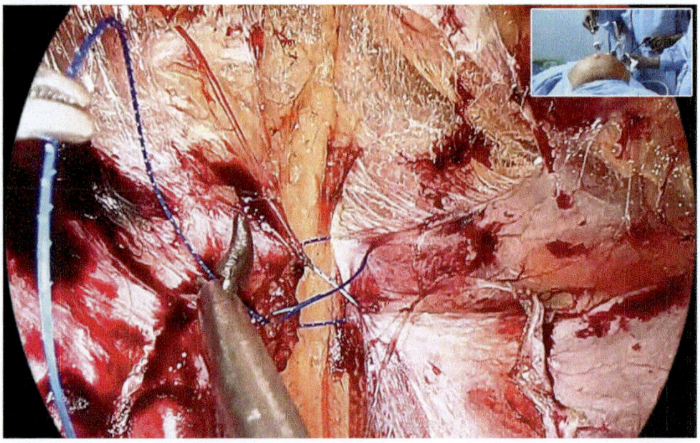

Fig. 12: Closing posterior rectus sheath.

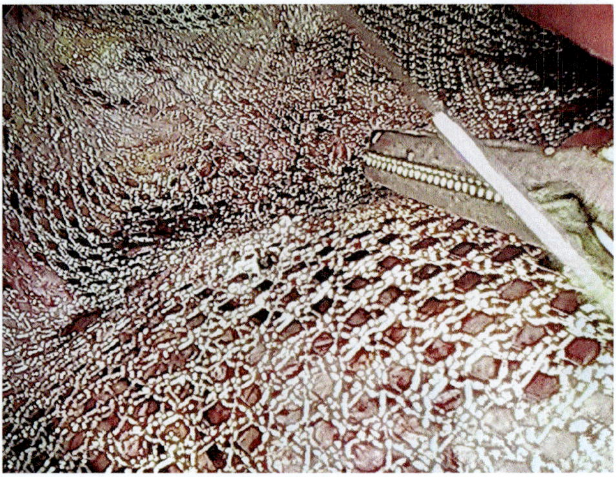

Fig. 13: Mesh placement.

Closure

After changing to a 5 mm telescope, fascia is closed at the 10 mm trocar site using a 0-polypropylene suture under vision using a cobbler needle. The 5 mm and 10 mm ports are closed with subcuticular skin sutures.

DIFFICULTIES WHICH WE USUALLY FACE DURING THE eTEP PROCEDURE

- During the introduction, the first trocar can go into the peritoneal cavity:
  - Convert and proceed with IPOM/IPOM Plus as it is very difficult to dissect the space when pneumoperitoneum is present.
  - Convert it to TARM repair, i.e., laparoscopic transabdominal retromuscular repair. In that case, a transverse incision is made at the level of the hernial defect, extending from the right linea semilunaris to the left linea semilunaris in the posterior rectus sheath. Standing between the legs of the patient, the upper aspect of the retrorectus space is dissected below upward. The cart is then shifted to the leg end of the patient. Standing on the left side of the patient, the lower retrorectus space is dissected above downward. The anterior rectus sheath defect is suture closed. A mesh is placed and the posterior defect is closed with the 0 V-Loc PBT suture.
- Lack of dissection space due to pneumoperitoneum
  - An additional trocar is placed into the peritoneal cavity and the peritoneal air can be let out so that more dissection space can be obtained.
- Bleeding
  - Control of bleeding with a bipolar
  - Saline wash
  - Pressure and mopping with gauze
  - Placing transfascial sutures (rare)
- During the dissection of linea alba, buttonholes may be made. Before keeping the mesh, all these buttonholes should be suture closed using 0-polypropylene or 0 V-Loc PBT suture.

ADVANTAGES OF EXTENDED TOTALLY EXTRAPERITONEAL REPAIR

A mesh can be placed outside the peritoneal cavity. The pain is much less as there are no tacks or transfascial fixation.

REFERENCES

1. Baig SJ, Priya P. Extended totally extraperitoneal repair (eTEP) for ventral hernias: Short-term results from a single centre. J Minim Access Surg. 2019;15(3):198-203.

2. Varacallo M, Scharbach S, Al-Dhahir MA. Anatomy, Anterolateral Abdominal Wall Muscles. [Updated 2023 Jul 24]. In: StatPearls [Internet]. Treasure Island (FL): StatPearls Publishing; 2023 Jan-. Available from: https://www.ncbi.nlm.nih.gov/books/NBK470334/
3. Jani K, Contractor S. Retrorectus sublay mesh repair using polypropylene mesh: cost-effective approach for laparoscopic treatment of ventral abdominal wall hernias. J Minim Access Surg. 2019;15(4):287-92. doi: 10.4103/jmas.JMAS_20_19. Erratum in: J Minim Access Surg. 2019 Jun 14;: Erratum in: J Minim Access Surg. 2019;15(4):362. PMID: 31031328; PMCID: PMC6839350.

Chapter 11

Laparoscopic Transabdominal Retromuscular Repair

INTRODUCTION

Various laparoscopic approaches were developed in the last three decades for managing ventral hernias. Intraperitoneal onlay mesh (IPOM) causes less tissue trauma, and outcomes are better when compared with open repair. Defect closure was needed for better regaining of muscle function and for preventing cupping of mesh (IPOM plus). The difficulties encountered were cost of the dual mesh, chance of adhesions due to intraperitoneal mesh, and pain due to use of tack or transfascial sutures. This was partially circumvented by placing a polypropylene mesh in the peritoneal cavity. Two modifications were developed to take care of these issues—extended totally extraperitoneal (eTEP) repair and transabdominal retromuscular (TARM) repair. The procedure of TARM repair was developed by Dr Ashwin A Masurkar.[1] TARM repair and eTEP had advantages of midline closure and combination of posterior component separation whenever necessary. These advantages were not there with transabdominal sublay mesh repairs reported initially.

PREOPERATIVE

General Anesthesia

Modified lithotomy position with leg split with the operation theater (OT) table flexed in the middle to provide extension of spine for a wider range of hand movements is recommended.

Nasogastric tube and urinary catheter placement should be checked.

PROCEDURE

Types of TARM repair procedure:

- Three-port TARM repair
- Six-port TARM repair
- TARM repair with transversus abdominis muscle release (TAR).

Three-port Transabdominal Retromuscular Repair

The first trocar placement is by modified Hasson technique or with an Optiview trocar under vision. The primary trocar is placed in the midline, suprapubic for upper abdominal defects. The trocar has to be slightly on the left side in the epigastrium for lower abdominal defects. Two working ports are placed on either side of the primary trocar. The trocar position is the same as in eTEP.

If adhesions are present, they are lysed and contents are reduced. A transverse incision is made about 5 cm proximal to the hernial defect, taking the peritoneum and posterior rectus sheath together. This is called peritoneum and posterior rectus sheath (PPRS) flap. This opens up retromuscular space, which is dissected from above downward or below upward. On reaching the hernial defect, the peritoneum needs to be divided, and dissection is proceeded. The lateral margin of the dissection will be 5 cm from the hernial margin.

Midline tissue suturing is performed using 0 V-Loc PBT (polybutylene terephthalate; Polybutester) suture 45 cm/15 cm. A 15 cm long thread may be sufficient to take three to five bites. For larger defects, we can use either a 45 cm long thread or multiple 15 cm long threads. An adequately sized polypropylene mesh is placed with 3–5 cm overlap. PPRS flaps are now closed with a 0 V-Loc PBT suture.

Port closure and postoperative care are same as those of IPOM.

Complications

Loss of vascularity of PPRS flap and mesh exposure to peritoneal cavity are the main complications. As far as possible, minimize the lateral dissection to avoid postoperative issues. For smaller hernias, do not dissect lateral to the inferior epigastric vessels.

Six-port Transabdominal Retromuscular Repair

Six-port TARM repair is preferred when the defect is larger lengthwise or there is associated divarication recti or when there are multiple midline defects. Three ports are placed in the lower abdomen and three ports in the upper abdomen. At the level of the umbilicus, a transverse incision is made on the abdominal wall from inside, extending from the right linea semilunaris to the left linea semilunaris. The PPRS flap is raised. The upper aspect of the retrorectus space is dissected below upward, the surgeon standing between the legs of the patient. The cart is then shifted to the leg end of the patient. Standing on the left side of the patient, the lower retrorectus space is dissected above downward. The anterior rectus sheath defect is closed with a 0 V-Loc PBT suture. A polypropylene mesh is placed. The PPRS defect is closed with a 0 V-Loc PBT suture **(Fig. 1)**.

Transabdominal Retromuscular Repair with Transversus Abdominis Muscle Release

Transabdominal retromuscular repair with TAR is performed if the hernial defect is so large that the sheath closure could not be achieved. This is also

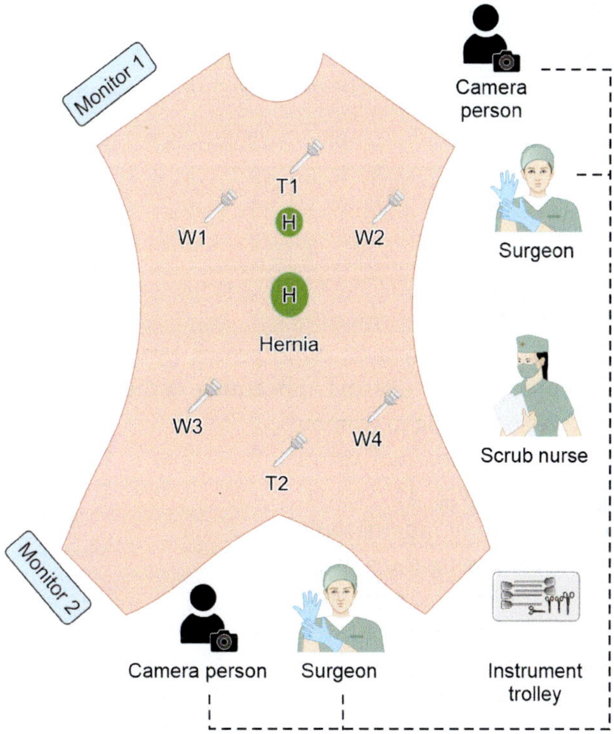

Fig. 1: Port positions of six-port transabdominal retromuscular (TARM) repair.

suited for lumbar hernias. The initial procedure is as in three-port TARM repair. The transverse incision is longer and crosses the linea semilunaris on one or both sides. Safeguarding the neurovascular bundles, TAR is performed. A larger polypropylene mesh is placed. During the suture closure, abdominal insufflation pressure can be reduced to 8 mm Hg so that the abdomen is relaxed.

REFERENCE

1. Masurkar AA. Laparoscopic trans-abdominal retromuscular (TARM) repair for ventral hernia: a novel, low-cost technique for sublay and posterior component separation. World J Surg. 2020;44(4):1081-5.

Chapter 12

Abdominoplasty with Concomitant Ventral Hernia Repair

INTRODUCTION

Abdominoplasty, also known as tummy-tuck procedure, is a surgical procedure to improve the shape and appearance of the abdomen.[1] Majority of ventral hernias occurring in women are associated with abdominal apron (hanging abdomen) **(Fig. 1)**. Ventral hernia repair by open or laparoscopic surgery means correcting the ventral hernia only. The excess skin and fat can be removed by combining dermolipectomy. It not only gives a better cosmesis, but also provides abdominal wall reconstruction so that the mesh stays on a firm surface and the chances of recurrence are lesser.

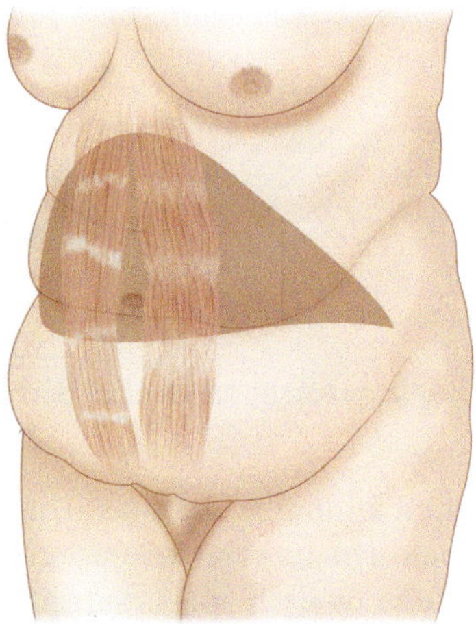

Fig. 1: Abdominal apron.

The first official abdominoplasty was performed by Drs Demars and Marx in France in 1890. In 1899, Kelly a gynecologic surgeon in Baltimore, Maryland, described the steps that we follow today.[2]

TYPES

Abdominoplasty can be of five types **(Fig. 2)**:[1]

1. Full abdominoplasty (traditional abdominoplasty)
2. Partial abdominoplasty (mini tuck for small aprons)
3. Lipoabdominoplasty (full abdominoplasty with liposuction for prominent love bands)
4. Extended abdominoplasty (belt lipectomy for anterior and posterior aprons)
5. Reverse abdominoplasty (for upper abdominal hanging with large hanging breasts).

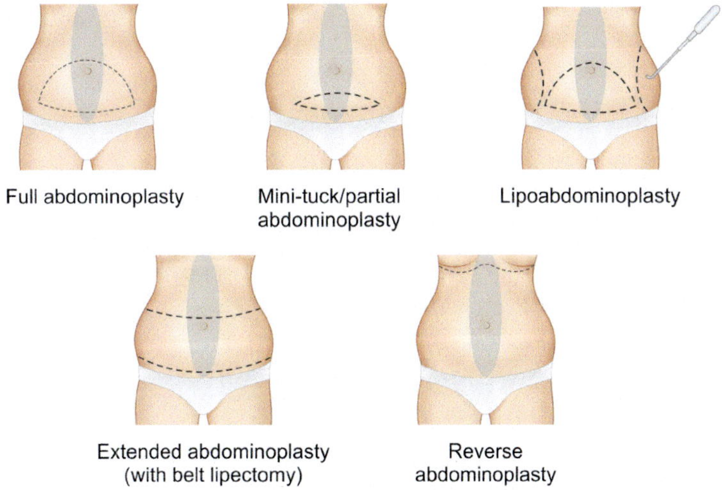

Fig. 2: Methods of abdominoplasty.

INDICATIONS

Excess fat and poor elasticity of the skin lead to weakened connective tissue of the abdomen, which forms a hanging abdomen (apron).

Causes

- Multiple pregnancies
- Multiple surgeries
- Obesity
- Significant weight loss
- Aging
- Natural body type

CONTRAINDICATIONS

- Absolute—severe cardiorespiratory failure, morbid obesity, and bleeding diathesis
- Relative—expecting mothers who have not completed family, uncontrolled diabetes mellitus, old age, and badly scarred abdomen where we may not get healthy skin to close.

STEPS (FIG. 3)

Preoperatively, cardiology and anesthesia fitness are taken, preoperative workup is completed, and ultrasound of the abdomen is done to rule out or detect any pathology which has to be tackled simultaneously. The patient is kept nil per oral for 6 hours. After part preparation, a microshield

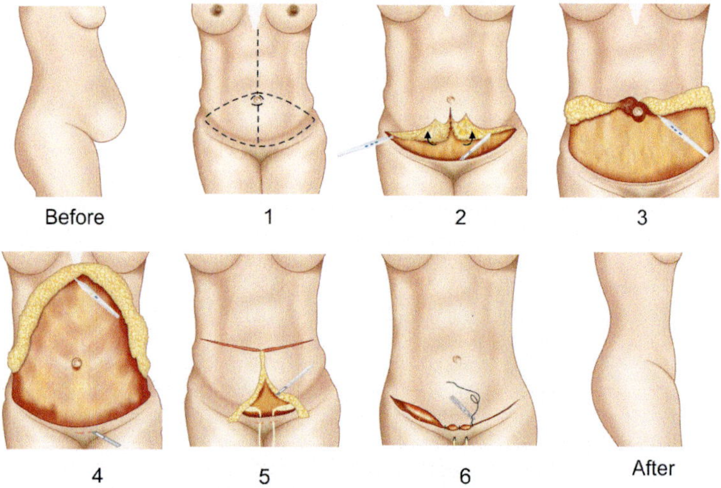

Fig. 3: Steps of abdominoplasty.

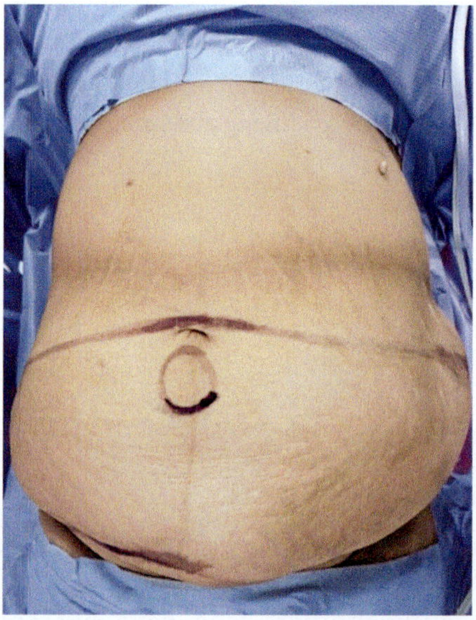

Fig. 4: Skin marking.

scrub bath is given. An informed consent is taken, especially mentioning neoumbilicus or umbilectomy. A microshield scrub bath is given on the day of the surgery also.

Site marking should be done in the room, clearly telling the patient the extent of scar in relation to their undergarments. The marking is done better in the standing position **(Fig. 4)**.

In operation theater at induction, one dose of antibiotic (Injection ceftriaxone + sulbactam 1.5 g for nonobese patients and 3 g for obese patients) is given. The patient is under general or regional anesthesia (spinal + epidural anesthesia) and painted and draped. He is placed at supine position with arms abducted 90°.

Incision and Flap Raising

A lower abdominal crease incision is made with a tongue in the midline with convexity toward the umbilicus **(Fig. 5)**. This may be removed later based on the length of the supraumbilical skin flap. The lateral extent of the incision is decided based on the lateral extent of the apron. The incision is deepened up to the rectus sheath, leaving a thin layer of areolar connective tissue above the sheath to preserve lymphatics.

The flap is raised superiorly up to the xiphisternum in the midline to rib margin in the lateral aspect **(Fig. 6)**. Both hypochondrial regions are not dissected as the perforating vessels at this region give vascularity to the flap. Inferiorly, the flap is raised up to pubic symphysis.

A vertical infraumbilical incision may be placed to ease the holding of upper flaps **(Fig. 7)**. The umbilicus can be either preserved or removed if it is badly scarred, thinned out because of hernia, or severely displaced in the apron. If the umbilicus is preserved, a good amount of the fat is retained around it to provide vascularity to the umbilicus.

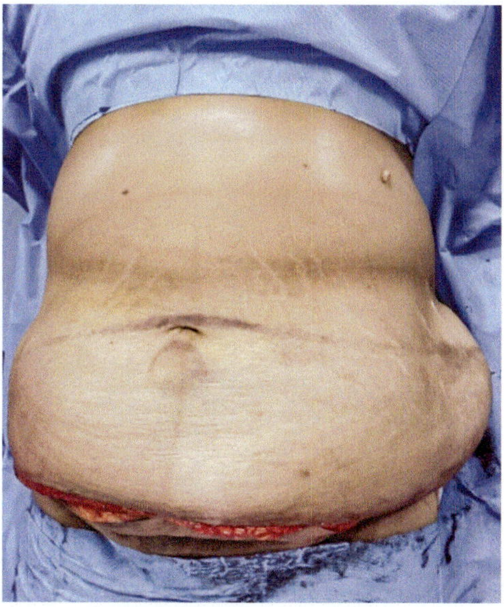

Fig. 5: Incision of skin.

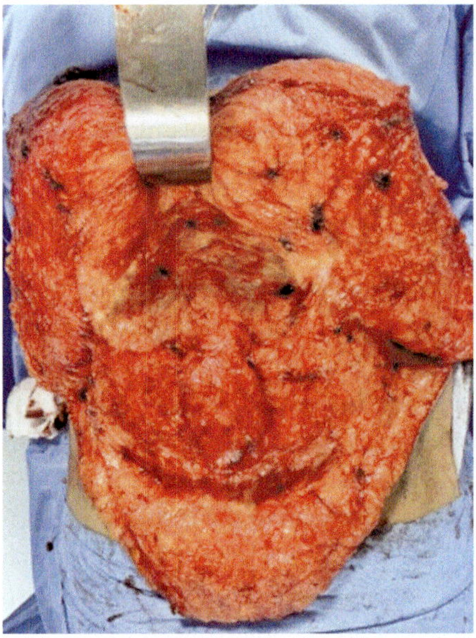

Fig. 6: Flap raising.

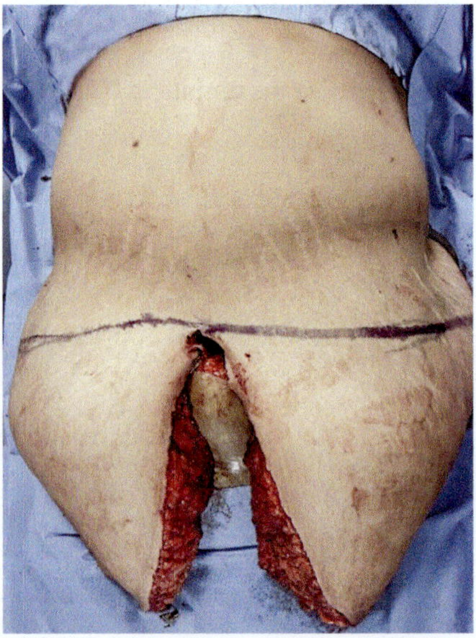

Fig. 7: Vertical infraumbilical incision.

Ventral Hernia Repair (Fig. 8)

The hernial defect in an abdominoplasty is repaired by open means with an onlay or a sublay mesh **(Fig. 9)**. Commonly, we perform open sublay

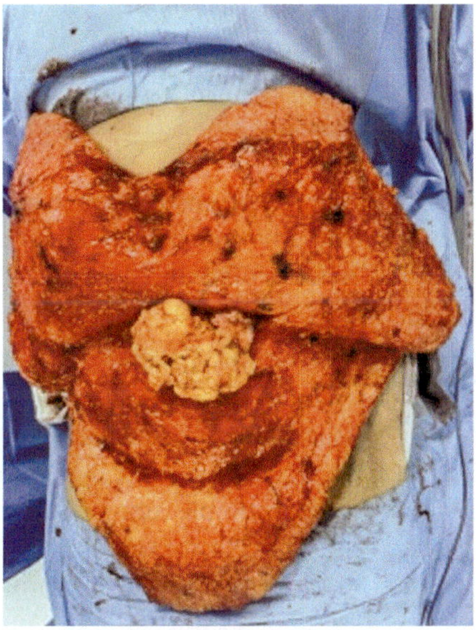

Fig. 8: Ventral hernia.

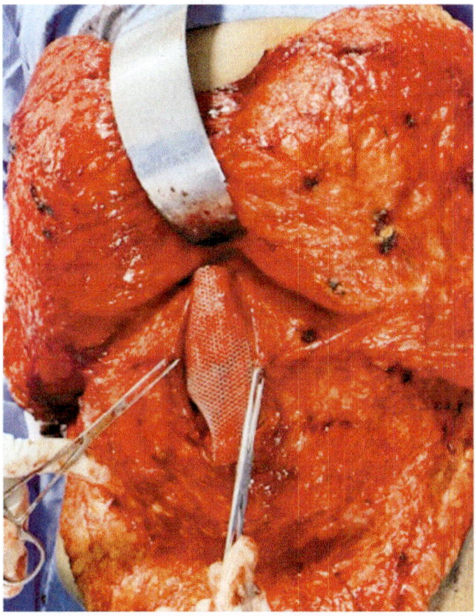

Fig. 9: Sublay mesh.

repair as it keeps the mesh away from the skin to lessen the mesh infection. Hernial contents are reduced, adhesiolysis is performed, and in case of huge hernias with omentum, omentectomy is done. Midline is closed with polypropylene 1-0 suture. The anterior rectus sheath is opened vertically on both sides to the entire length of the defect. The retrorectus space is dissected and an adequately sized polypropylene mesh is placed (generally 10 cm wide mesh) **(Fig. 10)**. Gentamicin 80 mg is instilled on the mesh. The rectus muscle is approximated, and the anterior rectus sheath is closed with a 1-0 polypropylene suture.

An alternate method is to open the posterior rectus sheath through the hernial defect. Then the retrorectus space is dissected, and the posterior rectus sheath is closed. The mesh is placed in the retrorectus space and the defect is closed **(Fig. 11)**.

Plication and Darning (Fig. 12)

A majority of the cases are associated with divarication of recti. This can be corrected by placing plication sutures followed by darning sutures on the rectus sheath. Plicating sutures are multiple running sutures with bites taken perpendicular to the suture line (similar to Keel's repair). In darning suture, each bite is taken parallel to the suture line in a figure-of-eight fashion. Darning sutures can be continuous or intermittent. All these sutures are taken with 1-0 polypropylene. Plication sutures are to crumble the excess rectus sheath to midline, and darning sutures are tension-free sutures for an additional hold. Based on the extent of divarication, darning and plication sutures are placed horizontally. Sutures are placed in the midline along the epigastric tunnel using vicryl 2-0 suture to prevent seroma. It also lessens the epigastric bulge.

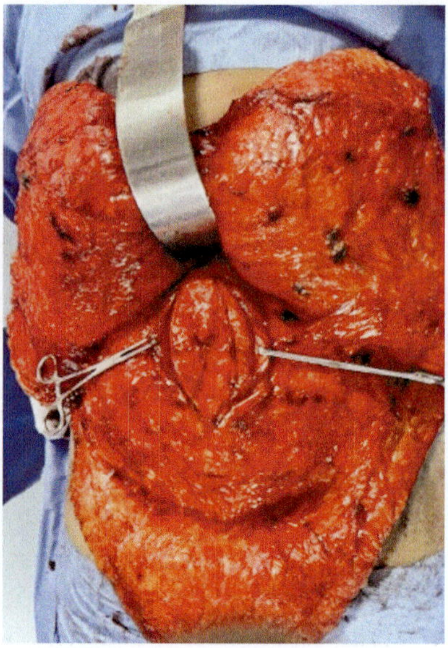

Fig. 10: Dissecting retrorectus space.

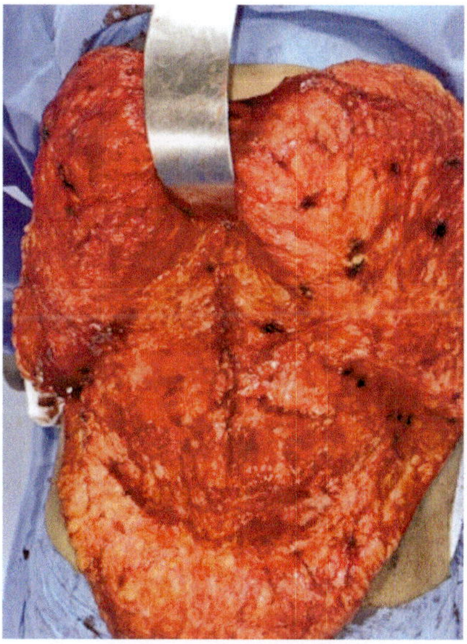

Fig. 11: Defect closure.

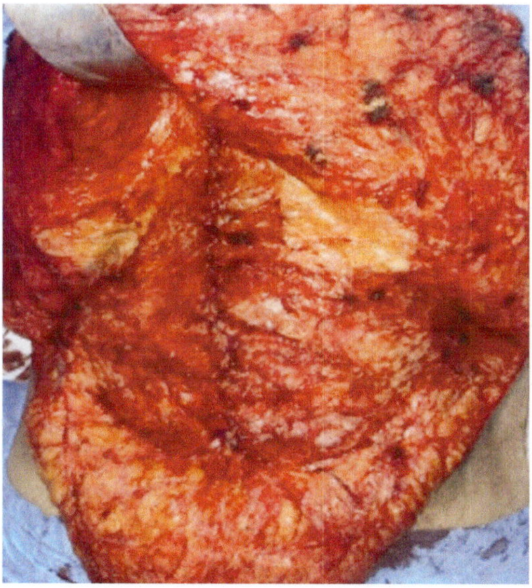

Fig. 12: Plication and darning.

Neoumbilicus/Umbilicus Transposition (Fig. 13)

In cases where the umbilicus is very deep, inflamed, and scarred or has an umbilical defect with thinned-out tissues, we may have to excise the

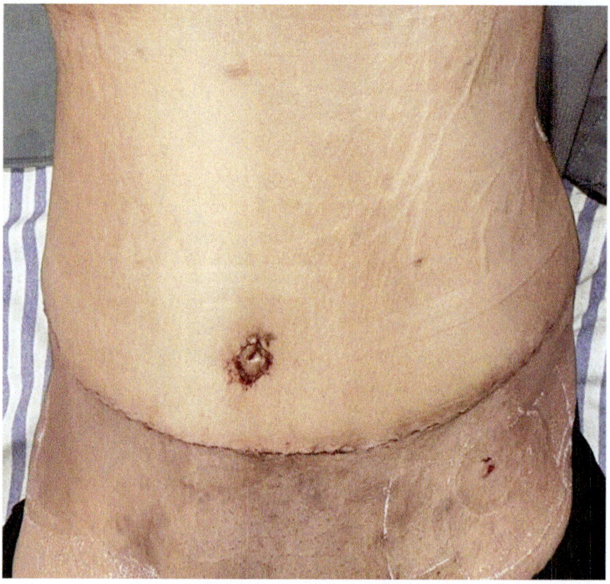

Fig. 13: Umbilicus transposition.

umbilicus and create a new one (neoumbilicus). The site for umbilicus is marked as a junction between the line joining both anterior superior iliac spine (ASIS) and midline.

Marking is made on the anterior rectus sheath along the midline just inferior to the skin marking. A curvilinear incision is given approximately 2 cm using a number 15 blade. The fat underlying this incision is excised (approximately 2 × 2 cm), leaving a small amount of subcutaneous fat for vascularity of the skin. The fat is held with Allis forceps and excised with monopolar. Three (Ethilon number 2-0) sutures are placed (one on the upper margin and two on the lateral angles of the incision), hitching the incision with the anterior rectus sheath.

Before the sutures are tied, a purse string suture is placed around the incision using 3-0 polydioxanone suture (PDS) and the knot is submerged. Ethilon sutures are tied into the anterior rectus sheath, while the assistant is pushing the newly made umbilicus down.

In cases where the umbilicus is healthy and viable, a 1 × 1 cm circular incision is made at a point marked on the skin where the umbilicus needs to come out. Ethilon sutures are placed hitching the skin of the incision and roof of the umbilicus on all four corners. The umbilicus is delivered and Ethilon sutures tied. The umbilicus is fashioned and skin closure is done using 3-0 monofilament absorbable suture. The stump of the umbilicus can be reduced by placing interrupted sutures.

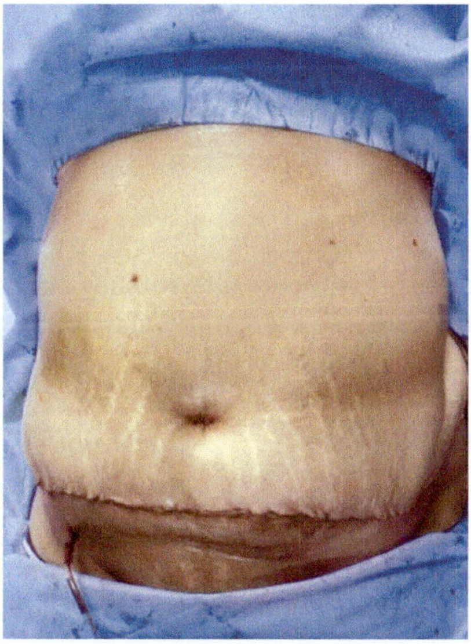

Fig. 14: Wound closure with a drain.

Dermolipectomy

The patient is positioned in head-up and legs-up position (Fowler's position). Maximum skin can be pulled and excised to ensure a tight closure. The excess suprapubic skin can be excised depending on the upper flap approximation. Never make a beveled cut to excise more of subcutaneous fat, as it may lead to flap necrosis. Subcutaneous fat can be hitched with anterior rectus sheath to lessen the seroma collection. A tube drain is placed under the subcutaneous fat and the closure of the wound can be done in layers by using a vicryl 2-0 suture; the skin can be closed by placing a subcuticular suture using monoglyde 3-0 suture **(Fig. 14)**. A sterile pressure dressing is applied on the wound.

POSTOPERATIVE CARE

- IV antibiotics and analgesics—tramadol, paracetamol, and diclofenac may be given. Tapentadol nasal spray, as and when needed
- Fowler's position
- Abdominal binder
- Thromboembolic deterrent (TED) stockings and deep vein thrombosis (DVT) pump
- Mobilization after 24 hours
- Small frequent meals
- Discharge on postoperative day (POD) 2/3
- Wound care

COMPLICATIONS

Seroma Formation

Drainage tubes in place after surgery can help reduce the risk of excess fluid. Seroma will be less if abdominal binder is applied postoperatively.

Scarring/Keloid

Scarring can be reduced by subcuticular stitches and application of scar-reducing ointments locally. Keloid can be managed by serial intrathecal steroid injections.

Changes in Skin Sensation

This usually diminishes in the months after the procedure.

Bleeding, Infection, and Anesthesia-related Problems

Like any other type of major surgery, a tummy tuck poses a risk of bleeding, infection, and anesthesia-related problems.

Abdominal Compartment Syndrome

Full abdominoplasty has the risk of causing abdominal compartment syndrome. This complication can be relieved by decompression of the abdominal wall.

Margin Necrosis

Minimal flap necrosis due to reduced vascularity is managed by aspirin/clopidogrel. If necrosis is larger, it may necessitate excision and secondary suturing.

REFERENCES

1. Regan JP, Casaubon JT. Abdominoplasty. [Updated 2023 Jul 24]. In: StatPearls [Internet]. Treasure Island (FL): StatPearls Publishing; 2023 Jan-. Available from: https://www.ncbi.nlm.nih.gov/books/NBK431058/.
2. Kelly HA (1899) Report of gynecological cases. Johns Hopkins Med J 10:197.

Chapter

13 Diaphragmatic Hernias in Adult

INTRODUCTION

Diaphragmatic hernias, post-traumatic or congenital, are rare varieties of internal hernias **(Fig. 1)**. Laparoscopic repair is being increasingly favored for the repair of these hernias because of minimum morbidity and less postoperative pain for the patient. Congenital hernias when manifest in the neonatal period, the only option may be open surgery—thoracic or abdominal. But when the hernia appears in adulthood, laparoscopy is the preferred treatment option. Thoracoscopy and robotic surgery are newer methods for treatment of diaphragmatic hernia in adults, but the efficacy is yet to be proven.

ANATOMY OF DIAPHRAGM

Diaphragm is a dome-shaped musculotendinous partition between the thorax and the abdomen. It arises from septum transversum, pleuroperitoneal membranes, mediastinum (dorsal mesentery of esophagus), and cervical myotomes. Structurally, the diaphragm consists of two parts, a central tendinous portion and a peripheral muscular portion. The muscular

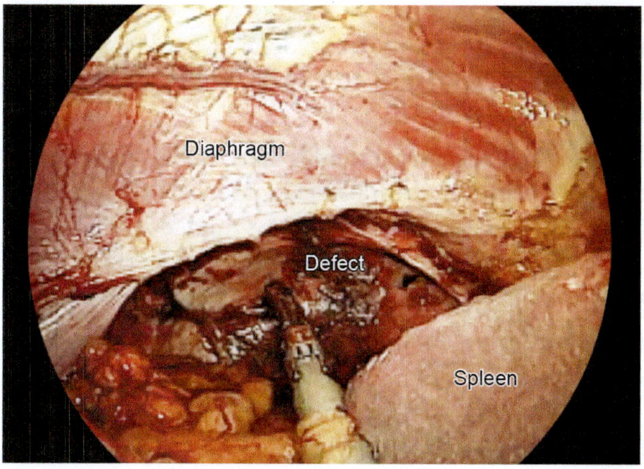

Fig. 1: Diaphragmatic hernia.

origin arises from lower six ribs bilaterally, the posterior of xiphoid process, external and internal arcuate ligaments, and the crura. It has openings for passage of inferior vena cava, esophagus, and aorta.[1]

CLASSIFICATION

Diaphragmatic hernia of adulthood is classified into two—congenital or acquired. Congenital hernias are posterolateral—Bochdalek hernia, parasternal—Morgagni-Larrey hernia, and peritoneopericardial hernias or eventration of diaphragm. Traumatic hernias are classified based on etiology into those due to penetrating trauma of the abdomen or those due to blunt abdominal trauma including unrecognized diaphragmatic rupture.[2] Diaphragmatic rupture mostly occurs on the left side as the right side is protected by the liver.

CLINICAL FEATURES

Diaphragmatic hernia of adulthood usually presents as postprandial chest discomfort or gastric outlet obstruction. The patients may have minor symptoms such as dyspepsia or epigastric pain. Occasionally, it is an incidental finding on X-ray of the chest, ultrasound scan of the abdomen, computed tomography (CT) scan of the thorax, or upper gastrointestinal endoscopy.

INDICATION OF LAPAROSCOPIC REPAIR

Presence of diaphragmatic hernia of adulthood.

CONTRAINDICATIONS[3]

- Unstable patient (absolute)
- Hernia >10 cm (relative)
- Hernial defect connecting into hiatal opening (relative).

LAPAROSCOPIC REPAIR

Preparation: Skin and hair preparation is done before shifting the patient to the operation theater (OT). Preanesthetic orders are followed. The patient is kept nil per oral for 8 hours before surgery. Antibiotic prophylaxis is given based on the hospital protocol, i.e., tobramycin—2 hours prior to surgery and ceftriaxone sulbactam at induction.

Anesthesia: General anesthesia.

POSITIONING THE PATIENT

After induction, the patient is kept in Lloyd Davies position with reverse Trendelenburg tilt (up to 30° head elevation). The patient is kept supine with legs apart to accommodate the operating surgeon. The first assistant stands on the left side and the second assistant (laparoscope operator) stands on the right side.

ENTRY AND TROCAR POSITIONING

A 10 mm trocar is placed slightly toward the left of midline, midway between the xiphoid process and the umbilicus. Open technique/Optiview-port technique is chosen based on the convenience of the surgeon. The bowel at the site of entry is inspected and tilt is given. Three or four additional ports are placed that are 5 or 3 mm, at right subcostal, right midclavicular, left midclavicular, and left anterior axillary line. The midclavicular ports are working ports for the operating surgeon, while the other ports are used to retract the liver, stomach, and greater omentum.

STEPS OF PROCEDURE

1. *Visualization of hernia defect:* In case of emergency laparoscopy for traumatic rupture, diagnostic laparoscopy has to be performed for identification of other injuries. The hernial defect is then located and the contents are reduced with atraumatic graspers. The adhesions between the contents and the hernial sac are lysed with sharp dissection using scissors or harmonic scalpel. If the neck of the sac is narrow, a small lateral cut is made to release the contents.
2. *Reduction of sac:* Surgeons differ in their opinion regarding reduction of the hernial sac. Some do it routinely to avoid a residual cyst in the thorax,[4] while others avoid it completely to avoid pneumomediastinum and its related cardiovascular complications.[4] In our center, we do not reduce the hernial sac.
3. *Closure of defect:* If the hernial defect is getting approximated without tension, it is closed with simple or horizontal mattress sutures with 0 or number 1 nonabsorbable braided sutures. While taking sutures, you should be careful about the depth of the puncture so that the thoracic contents that are situated on the other side of the diaphragm are not injured. When the last suture is being tied, the air inside the sac is sucked out to avoid a residual cyst in the thorax.
4. *Placement of chest tube:* It is also controversial whether to place routinely a chest tube or not. Some do it always, while we prefer to be without a chest tube, and it is placed only if there is pneumothorax or lung injury. A thoracostomy set is kept ready for use so that in case of emergency, a rapid implantable cardioverter defibrillator (ICD) placement could be done.
5. *Prosthetic material placement:* If the defect is >3 cm, a prosthetic material should be used to reinforce the closure to prevent recurrence of hernia.

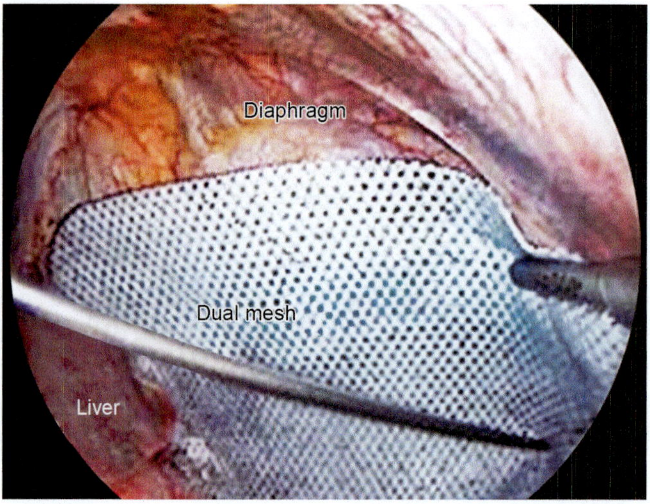

Fig. 2: Mesh placement.

Either a polypropylene mesh[5] or a composite mesh can be used[6] for reinforcement. It should cover at least 3–4 cm from the margin all around the defect.

6. *Fixation of the mesh:* This could be done with nonabsorbable sutures or tacks. Care should be taken during placement to avoid intrathoracic injury **(Fig. 2)**.

POSTOPERATIVE CARE

Postoperative chest X-ray is taken to look for pneumothorax. Oral sips are started once the patient recovers from anesthesia. Gradually, they are switched over to soft diet once the ileus subsides and the patient is discharged in 2–3 days. All routine activities can be resumed in a week's time and strenuous exercise in 2 weeks' time.

REFERENCES

1. Schumpelick V, Steinau G, Schluper I, Prescher A. Surgical embryology and anatomy of the diaphragm with surgical applications. Surg Clin North Am. 2000;80:213-39.
2. Rasiah KK, Crowe PJ. Laparoscopic repair of a traumatic diaphragmatic hernia. J Laprarosc Endosc Surg. 1995;5:405-7.
3. Mathews BD, Bui H, Harold KL, Kercher KW, Adrales A, Park A, et al. Laparoscopic repair of traumatic diaphragmatic injuries. Surg Endosc. 2003;17:254-8.
4. Newman L, Eubanks S, Bridges WM, Lucas G. Laparoscopic diagnosis and treatment of Morgagni hernia. Surg Laparosc Endosc. 1995;5:27-31.

5. Vrijland WW, Jeekel J, Steyerberg EW, Hoed PTD, Bonjer HJ. Intraperitoneal polypropylene mesh repair of incisional hernia is not associated with enterocutaneous fistula. Br J Surg. 2000;87:348-52.
6. Schnieder R, Herington JL Jr, Ganada AM. Marlex mesh in repair of diaphragmatic defect later eroding into the distal esophagus and stomach. Am Surg. 1979;45:337-9.

Chapter

14 Laparoscopic Hiatus Hernia Repair

INTRODUCTION

Gastroesophageal reflux disease is an extremely common disorder. It is estimated that 10% of the general population have hiatus hernia. In this chapter, we discuss about the indications for surgical treatment and also the role of laparoscopy in curing this disorder.

DEFINITION

Hiatus hernia is defined as a protrusion of any abdominal structure other than the esophagus into the thoracic cavity through a widening of the hiatus of the diaphragm.

CLASSIFICATION

Hiatus hernia is classified into the following subtypes:[1]

- *Type I:* Sliding hiatus hernia: Gastroesophageal junction migrates above the diaphragm. Fundus remains below the gastroesophageal junction.
- *Type II:* Pure paraesophageal hernias: The gastroesophageal junction remains in its normal position, while the fundus of the stomach herniates through the diaphragmatic hiatus adjacent to the esophagus.
- *Type III:* Combination of types I and II, where both gastroesophageal junction and fundus of stomach herniate.
- *Type IV:* Colon or small bowel may be the content.

95% of hiatal hernias are type I (sliding). The other varieties, types II, III, and IV (paraesophageal), are rare.

ETIOLOGY

Herniation occurs due to weakening of phrenoesophageal ligament due to depletion of elastin fibers. This leads to stretching of the ligament and proximal displacement of the gastroesophageal junction.

DIAGNOSIS

- On a plain chest X-ray, retrocardiac air–fluid level is seen in patients with paraesophageal hernia.

- On contrast-enhanced computed tomography (CECT) of the abdomen, hernial contents can be clearly assessed. Strangulation and intestinal obstruction could clearly be visualized on CECT.
- Upper gastrointestinal endoscopy allows visualization of mucosa of esophagus, stomach, and duodenum. The presence of esophagitis or Barrett's esophagus can also be detected.
- Esophageal manometry demonstrates the level of diaphragmatic crura and lower esophageal sphincter, and thus gives the size of the sliding component.
- pH testing confirms the presence of gastroesophageal reflex.

INDICATIONS FOR SURGERY[2]

- Types II, III, and IV—if symptomatic, should be repaired
- Elective repair of types II, III, and IV hernias that are completely asymptomatic is based on patient's age, other comorbidities, and chance of complications
- Type I hernia with reflux disease proven by pH monitoring or endoscopic evidence, i.e., Barrett's esophagus or erosive esophagitis, surgery is an option
- Acute gastric volvulus.

SYMPTOMATOLOGY

- Heartburn and reflux symptoms
- Postprandial fullness of chest/shortness of breath
- Respiratory symptoms due to pulmonary compromise and reduced functional vital capacity, aspiration pneumonia
- Esophageal ulceration and upper gastrointestinal bleed
- Iron deficiency anemia
- Obstructive symptoms such as dysphagia and postprandial fullness of chest.

PREDICTORS OF OUTCOME

- Obese patients have a higher chance of recurrence.
- The larger the defect, the higher the chance of recurrence.
- Elderly patients and those with comorbidities have a higher morbidity than younger patients.

LAPAROSCOPIC TECHNIQUE FOR HIATUS HERNIA REPAIR

Laparoscopy is the preferred option for hiatus hernia repair today. It has reduced morbidity and hospital stay. It is as effective as transabdominal open repair.

Preparation of the Patient

Patients are kept on overnight fasting and skin preparation is done as with any other laparoscopic procedure. Antibiotics are given as per hospital protocol.

Anesthesia

General anesthesia is used.

Positioning the Patient

Semilithotomy position/supine position with legs apart and arms tucked by the side of the patient is followed. The table is given reverse Trendelenburg tilt. The patient is firmly secured to the table and appropriately padded. The stomach is decompressed with a Ryle's tube.

Positioning of Equipment

The cart is placed at the head end of the patient. The surgeon stands in between the legs of the patient. The first assistant stands on the left of the surgeon and the camera assistant stands on the right of the surgeon.

Instrumentation

0° and 30° laparoscope, atraumatic tissue holders and dissectors (Babcock type and DeBakey type), atraumatic liver retractor, ultrasonic coagulation devices or electrosurgical equipment, and needle holder are the instruments used.

Port Placement

A 10–12 mm camera port is placed 15 cm below xiphisternum toward the left of midline to avoid the falciform ligament coming into view **(Fig. 1)**. It is placed by the open cut-down technique or direct entry using Optiview or safety trocars.

Two 5 mm working ports are placed on either side of the surgeon and the other two 5 mm ports are placed still laterally for liver retraction on the right side and for the first assistant on the left side.

Dissection of Hiatus

The liver is retracted to the right and the gastroesophageal junction is held by the assistant and retracted to the left. The left hand of the surgeon holds the lesser omentum, and it is divided longitudinally using an energy device held in the right hand of the surgeon **(Fig. 2)**. Division starts above the hepatic branches of the vagus and dissection continues till the right crus of diaphragm is seen clearly. The phrenoesophageal membrane is then divided. Posterior

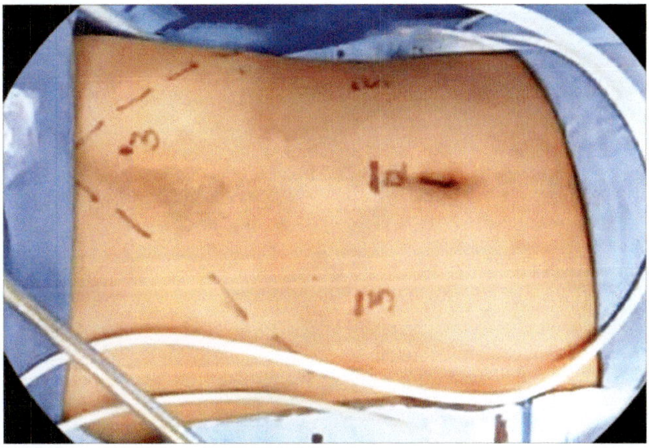

Fig. 1: Port placement.

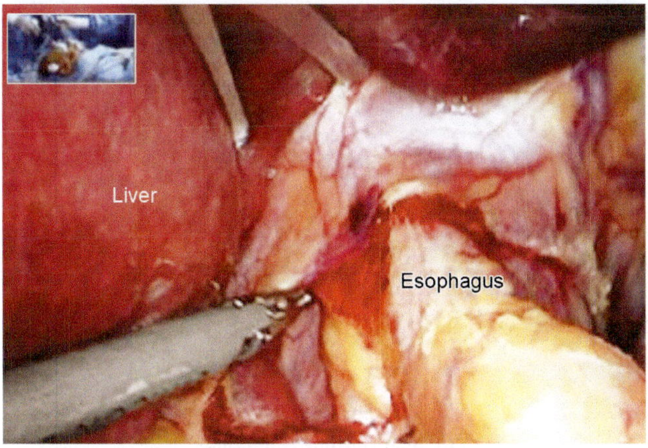

Fig. 2: Dissection of lesser omentum.

vagus is clearly seen now. Dissection is continued, separating esophagus medially and the right crus laterally till the origin of both crura is identified. Gastric fundus is pulled inferiorly and gastrophrenic omentum is divided. Dissection is continued anterior to the esophagus, pushing it posteriorly and thus separating it from the crural arch. Anterior vagus now comes into vision, and dissection is continued cephalad to separate esophagus from pleura and aorta and lateral crural attachments.

Mobilization of Fundus

Greater omentum is divided 10–15 cm down the cardiac notch by dividing the short gastric vessels with an energy device **(Fig. 3)**. During dissection, the surgeon pulls the stomach to the right side with an instrument, while the

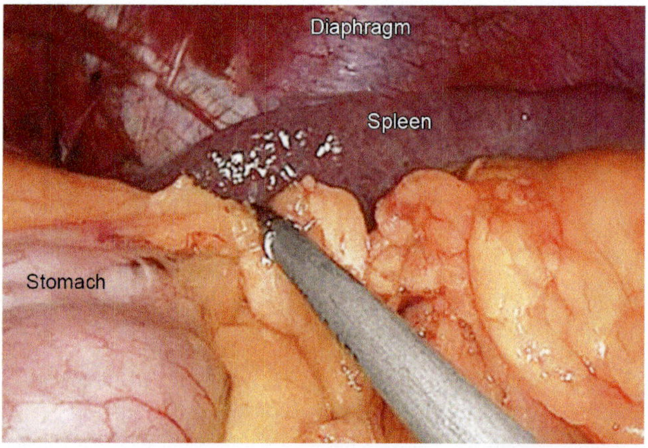

Fig. 3: Dividing the short gastric vessels.

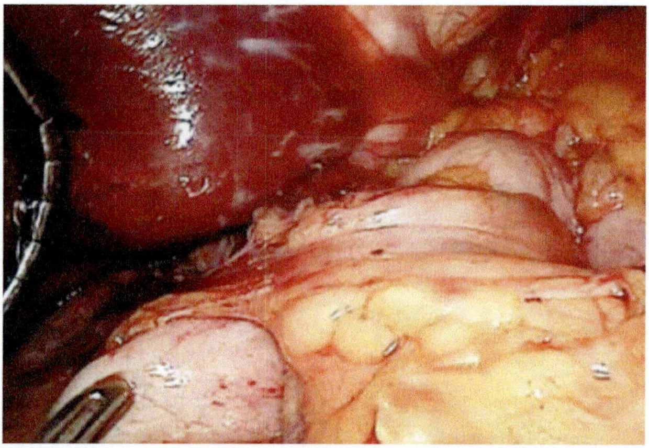

Fig. 4: Shoeshine maneuver.

assistant pulls the gastrosplenic omentum laterally. Thus, the entire fundus is mobilized and the dissected area on the right side is reached. Thus, the entire esophagus is mobilized from the hiatus.

Three things to be checked at this point of surgery are as follows.

1. The fundus is wrapped posterior to the esophagus by holding it with a left-hand instrument that is passed posterior to the esophagus. It is then released and thus tension is checked. If it retracts, more of the fundus is to be mobilized.
2. *Shoeshine maneuver:* This is done by moving back and forth the leading edge of the fundus by holding it on either side of esophagus. It is done to exclude rotation of fundus **(Fig. 4)**.
3. A minimum of 3.5 cm of the esophagus is to be maintained in the abdomen.

Approximation of Crura (Fig. 5)

Traction is maintained around esophagus using Penrose drain or even holding on to the wrap. Crura are then approximated using one or more sutures with 0-nonabsorbable braided polyester sutures. If the sutures are found to be under tension, they can be reinforced by keeping a polyester mesh. Adequacy of the hiatus is checked by keeping the instrument between the crura and the esophagus without force **(Fig. 6)**.

Fundoplication

The fundus, which is already wrapped around the esophagus, is now kept in position with the help of several interrupted sutures with

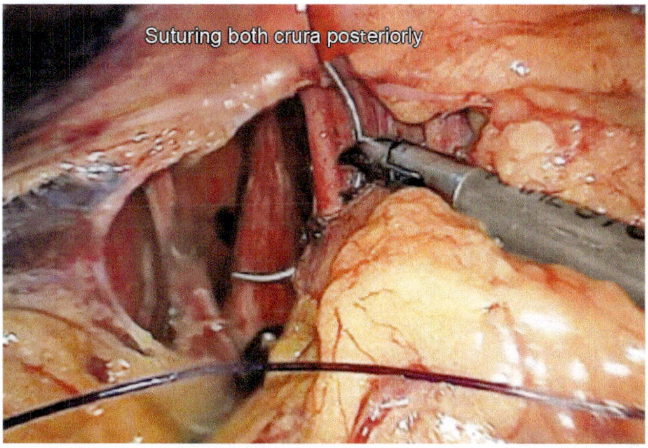

Fig. 5: Approximation of crura.

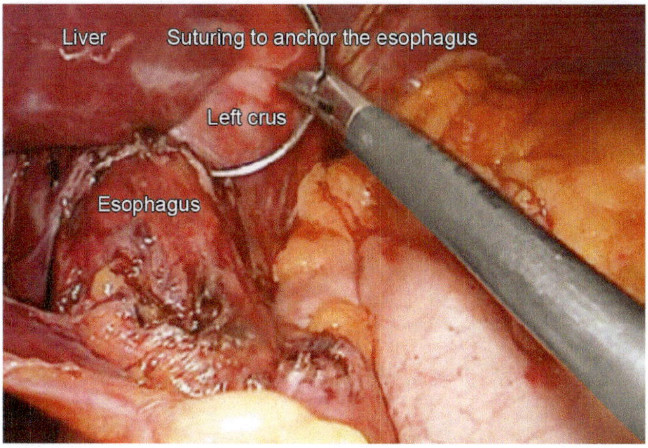

Fig. 6: Anchoring the esophagus.

0/2-0 nonabsorbable braided sutures. Sutures are taken from fundus on either side of the esophagus to the right of anterior vagus. Sutures are tied and tightened over a 50 or 60 French bougie in the esophagus. Care should be taken to observe that the wrap is made around the esophagus and not the stomach. The pad of fat at the angle of His helps to identify the gastroesophageal junction. Instead of 360° wrap as explained earlier, 270° wrap may be used if there is associated motility disorder. One set of sutures are taken from the esophagus at 11 o'clock position and approximated with fundus on the right side, and the next set of sutures is taken at 1 o'clock position of the esophagus and sutured with fundus on the left side of it. The fundus is then approximated with the right crus of diaphragm to prevent displacement of the wrap into the thoracic cavity **(Figs. 7 and 8)**.

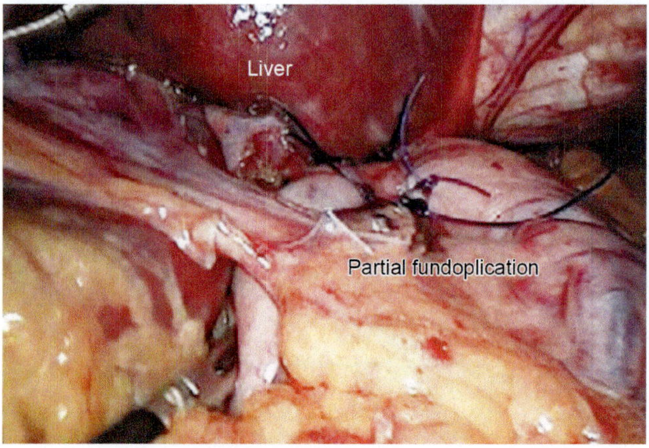

Fig. 7: Partial fundic wrap.

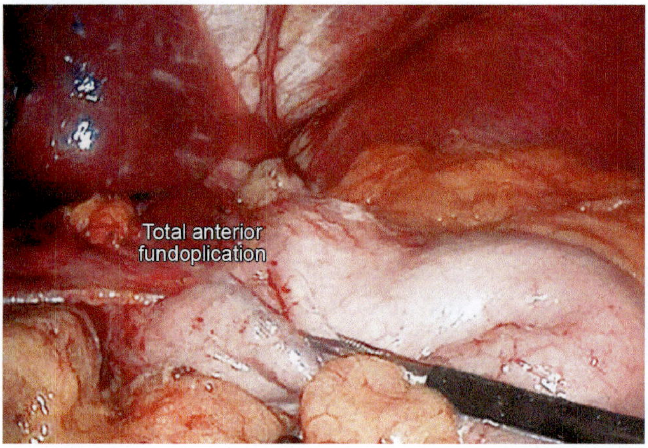

Fig. 8: Total fundoplication.

POSTOPERATIVE MANAGEMENT

Clear liquids are started a day after the surgery. Full liquid diet is started and is continued for 2–4 weeks. After 2 weeks, soft diet is started. A sudden increase in abdominal pressure predisposes to anatomical failure of fundoplication and hiatal hernia repair. Postoperative nausea and vomiting should be treated aggressively.

REFERENCES

1. Cha RR. Find out the differences by types of hiatal hernia! J Neurogastroenterol Motil. 2020;26(1):4-5.
2. Smith RE, Shahjehan RD. Hiatal Hernia. [Updated 2023 Aug 14]. In: StatPearls [Internet]. Treasure Island (FL): StatPearls Publishing; 2023 Jan-. Available from: https://www.ncbi.nlm.nih.gov/books/NBK562200/

Chapter

15 Pediatric Hernia Repair

MINIMAL INVASIVE INGUINAL HERNIA REPAIR IN CHILDREN

Open herniotomy is a time-tested procedure for inguinal hernia repair in children. Now studies are coming out with results in favor of laparoscopic hernia repair in children. Laparoscopic repair is fast becoming the gold standard for the treatment of inguinal hernia in children. The laparoscopic technique has the advantage that it is simple, feasible, and safe. Laparoscopic inguinal hernia repair in children was first described by Montupet in 1993, as noted by Schier.[1,2]

Preoperative Antibiotics

We give a single dose of third-generation cephalosporin, cefotaxime, at a dose of 35 mg/kg/dose. Most of the studies are in favor of a single dose of preoperative antibiotics to prevent wound infection. The child should be encouraged to empty the bladder prior to the procedure.

Anesthesia

Anesthesia is one area where you should not compromise when dealing with pediatric inguinal hernia. Always get an anesthesiologist who is well experienced and confident in giving pediatric anesthesia. Keep in mind the old saying that children are not small adults. Their physiology is different, and hypothermia is an important risk factor when dealing with the pediatric age group. Intraperitoneal gas pressure should be strictly monitored and kept between 8 and 10 mm Hg. The general principle is that it should not go above the portal pressure. We perform the procedure under general anesthesia. Postoperative pain can be reduced by giving caudal anesthesia along with general anesthesia. We undertake laparoscopic repairs for all children more than 6 months of age.[3-5]

Position

The procedure is performed with the child in supine position. A monitor is placed at the foot end toward the right side of the child. Surgeon, camera person, and scrub nurse are on the left side of the child.[3]

Operative Steps

Step 1: Port Placement

A 5-mm camera port is placed through a transumbilical incision. We start with "0°" scope and later change it to "30°" scope. Two additional working ports are placed in the midclavicular line just below the umbilicus on either side. These are preferably 3 mm ports. Since the abdominal wall is thin and the intra-abdominal pressure is kept low, the working ports should be placed carefully under vision.

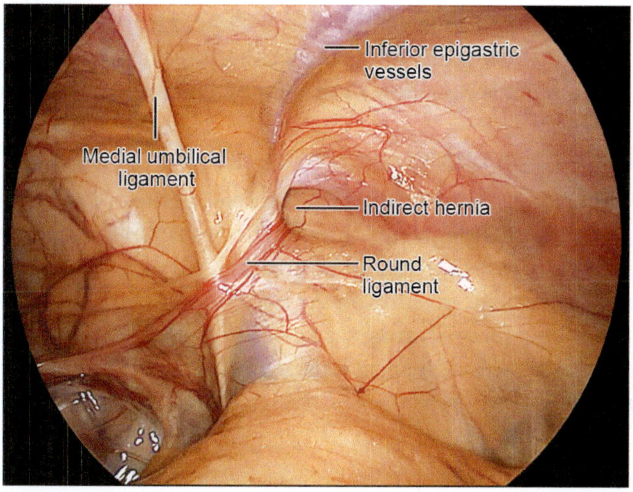

Fig. 1: Anatomical landmarks—right side, indirect defect, female child.

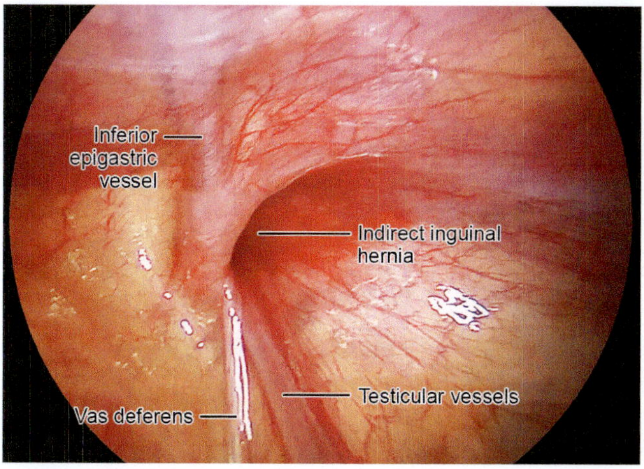

Fig. 2: Anatomical landmarks—right side, indirect defect, male child.

Step 2: Inspection of Abdominal Cavity

The entry point is inspected first. The table is positioned conveniently. After changing to "30°" scope, hernial orifices are inspected and the findings are confirmed. This is one area where laparoscopic repair clearly has an advantage over open repair. We can inspect the contralateral side, and if hernia is present, we can repair it in the same sitting **(Figs. 1 and 2)**.

Step 3: Division of Peritoneum

Peritoneum over the deep ring is divided circumferentially either with an energy source or with scissors. You should be careful not to injure the vas and testicular vessels in males. In females, the round ligament can be divided during dissection without any consequences. On the lateral aspect of the deep ring, the peritoneum is cut a little deeper for better closure **(Figs. 3 and 4)**.

Step 4: Suturing the Defect

We use 2-0 polydioxanone for suturing the defect. One of the 3 mm ports is removed, and a needle is inserted through the port site with a needle holder. Purse string sutures are taken from the proximal cut end of peritoneum near the deep ring at 2 o'clock position on the right side and 10 o'clock position on the left side without incorporating vas and testicular vessels **(Figs. 5 and 6)**. If contralateral processus vaginalis is patent, it is repaired. The needle is taken out through the 3 mm port site.

Step 5: Closure

The umbilical port is closed with 2-0 vicryl. 3 mm ports are not closed. The position of testis is always confirmed before completing the procedure.

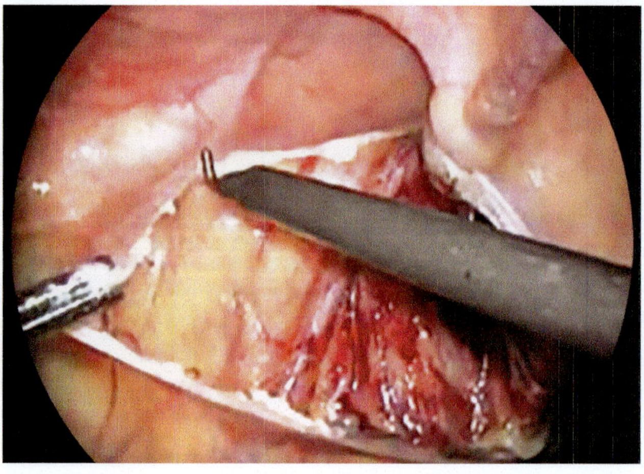

Fig. 3: Dividing peritoneum near the deep ring.

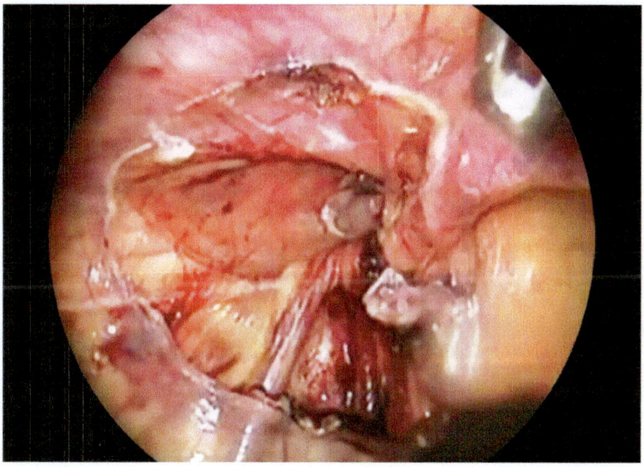

Fig. 4: Division of peritoneum completed.

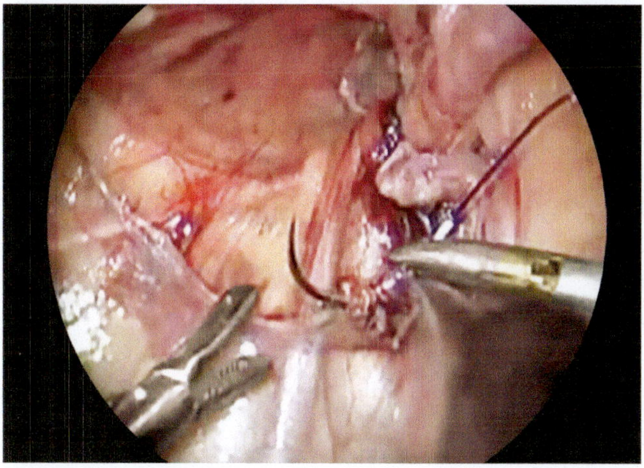

Fig. 5: Taking purse-string sutures.

MINIMAL INVASIVE OPEN PROCEDURE

Operative Steps

Step 1: Incision

A 1 cm incision is made in the inguinal region just lateral to pubic tubercle along the skin crease. The subcutaneous tissue is divided. External oblique aponeurosis is identified and nicked. The tissue dissections are done after a monopolar cautery application over a small area and then split by an artery forceps **(Figs. 7 and 8)**.

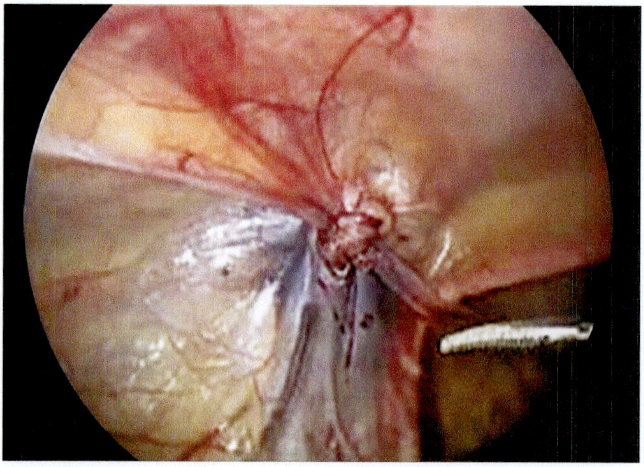

Fig. 6: Hernial defect closed.

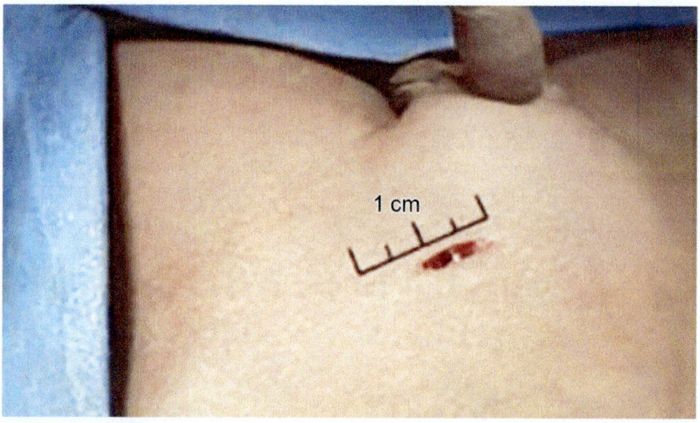

Fig. 7: Incision.

Step 2: Herniotomy

Retractors are pulled down and in toward the pubic tubercle. The inguinal ligament is identified **(Figs. 9 to 12)**. The sac appears as a white glistening structure, which is hooked up with a mosquito forceps. The cord structures are carefully dissected from the sac. The sac is opened and the neck is closed using 4-0 vicryl. The distal end is left open. In females, the broad ligament is divided and sutured along with the sac.

Step 3: Closure

The incision is closed in three layers, one stitch for external oblique and one for the subcutaneous tissue. The skin is closed with interrupted subcuticular suture **(Fig. 13)**.

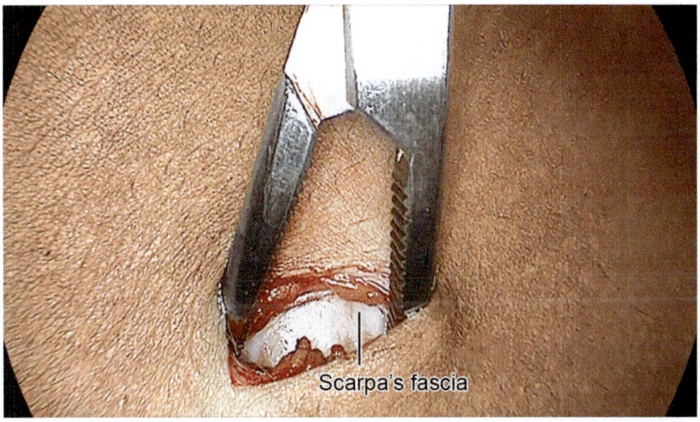

Fig. 8: Dissecting superficial fascial layer.

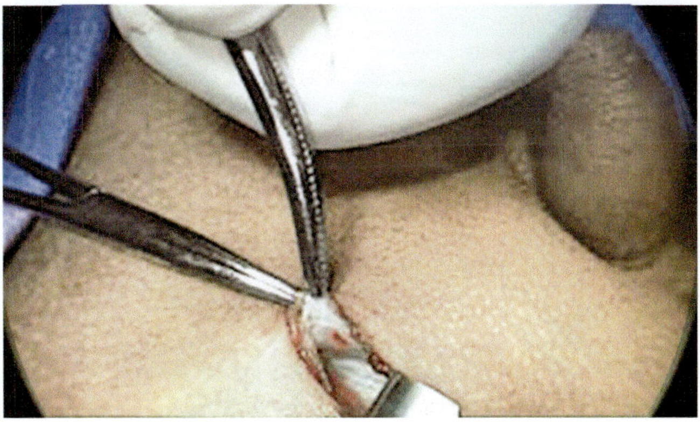

Fig. 9: Identifying inguinal ligament.

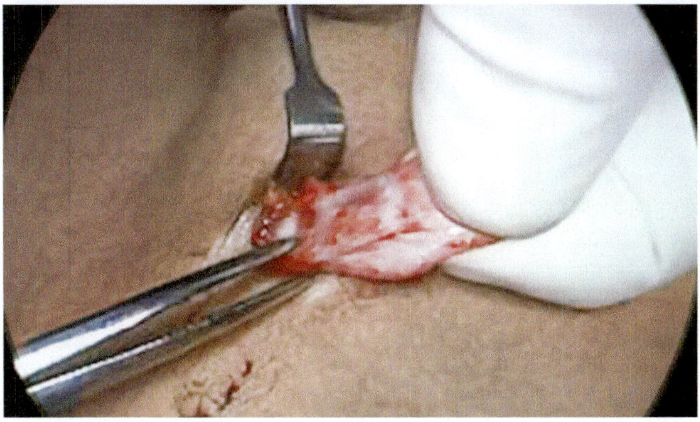

Fig. 10: Delivering the hernial sac.

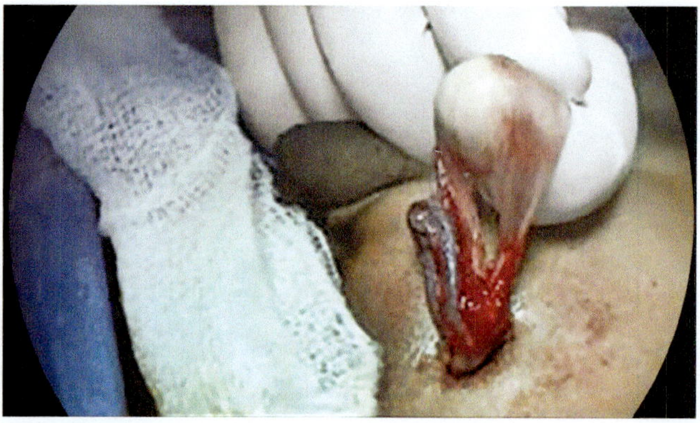

Fig. 11: Dissecting the hernial sac from cord structures.

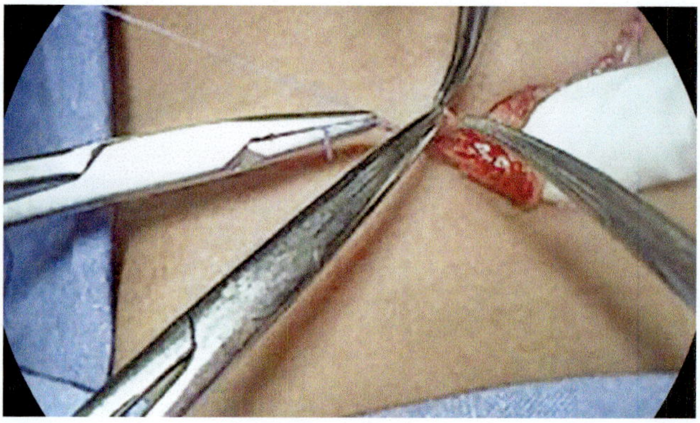

Fig. 12: Herniotomy.

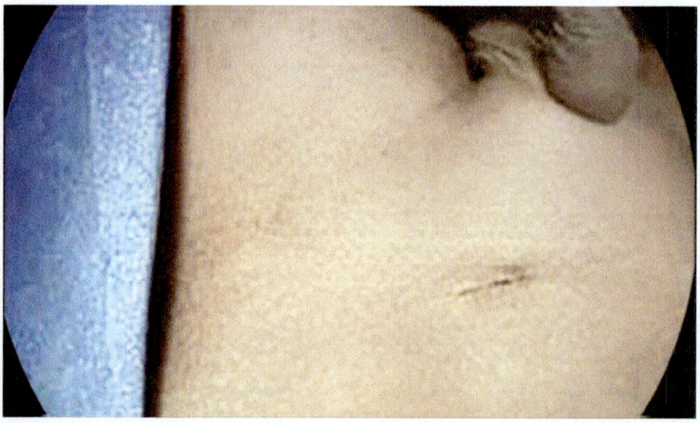

Fig. 13: Sutured wound.

ADVANTAGES OF LAPAROSCOPIC HERNIA REPAIR

- In laparoscopy, we can always examine the contralateral side and do the repair if needed and thus can avoid a procedure in future.[6,7]
- In bilateral cases, it is always preferable to do laparoscopic repair because the procedure can be performed through the same ports, whereas a second incision is mandatory in an open repair. In bilateral cases, operative time is less in laparoscopy as compared to open repair.[8]
- We can clearly see and safeguard vas and testicular vessels, which are less manipulated in laparoscopic repair as compared to open herniotomy. Chance of testicular atrophy and iatrogenic ascent of testis is very rare in laparoscopic repair.[8,9]
- In case of a female child with bilateral inguinal hernia, laparoscopy always helps to rule out any disorders of sexual differentiation.
- If there is an associated undescended testis, laparoscopy helps to confirm the diagnosis, and we can proceed with definitive management like orchiopexy.
- Other rare types of hernias such as femoral hernia or direct hernia can be detected and managed in the same sitting.[1,3,10]
- Since we are dividing the peritoneum, the chance for distal hydrocele is very less.[3]
- Decreased pain and fast recovery[3]
- Better cosmesis[3,8]
- Easy alternative in incarcerated, obstructed, sliding indirect hernias and recurrent hernias as inspection of contents possible. Laparoscopy avoids difficult dissection of edematous sac.[3,11]

DIFFICULTIES OF LAPAROSCOPIC HERNIA REPAIR

Those Directly Related to Laparoscopy

- Learning curve is more as it needs expertise for suturing in a child with smaller space for instrument movement.[4]
- Vascular injuries, bowel injury, and problems with pneumoperitoneum though reported are very rare.

Those Related to Hernia Repair

- Postoperative hydrocele—seen in laparoscopic procedure performed without dividing the peritoneum, though not of much significance[3]
- Very rare chance of injury to vas and testicular vessels, so always lift the peritoneum and then divide[9]
- Recurrence—reported rate is 0–5%, comparable to that of open repair.[1,4]

REFERENCES

1. Esposito C, St Peter SD, Escolino M, Juang D, Settimi A, Holcomb 3rd GW. Laparoscopic versus open inguinal hernia repair in paediatric patients: a systematic review. J Laparoendosc Adv Surg Tech A. 2014;24(11):811-8.
2. Schier F. Laparoscopic herniorrhaphy in girls. J Pediatr Surg. 1998;33:1495-7.
3. Grosfeld JL, Engum SA, Tam PKH. Hernias in children. In: Spitz L, Koran AG (Eds). Operative Paediatric Surgery, 7th edition. Boca Raton: CRC Press; 2013. pp. 277-99.
4. Glick PL, Boalanger SC. Inguinal hernias and hydroceles. In: Coran AG (Ed). Paediatric Surgery, 7th edition. Philadelphia: Elsevier Saunders; 2012. pp. 985-1001.
5. Landsman IS, Hays SR, Karsanae CJ, Franklin A. Paediatric Anesthesia. In: Coran AG (Ed). Paediatric Surgery, 7th edition. Philadelphia: Elsevier Saunders; 2012. pp. 201-26.
6. Yang C, Zhang H, Pu J, Mei H, Zheng L, Tong Q. Laparoscopic vs. open herniorrhaphy in the management of paediatric inguinal hernia: a systematic review and meta-analysis. J Pediatr Surg. 2011;46:1824-34.
7. Holcomb GW III, Miller KA, Chaignaud BA, Shew SB, Ostlie DJ. The parental perspective regarding the contralateral inguinal region in a child with a known unilateral inguinal hernia. J Pediatr Surg. 2004;39:480-2.
8. Shalaby R, Ibrahem R, Shahin M, Yehya A, Abdalrazek M, Alsayaad I, et al. Laparoscopic hernia repair versus open herniotomy in children: a controlled randomized study. Minim Invasive Surg. 2012:484135.
9. Oak S, Parelkar S, Agarwal P, Sailukar M, Gera P, Pathak R, et al. Laparoscopic surgery of inguinal hernia in children—experience with 110 repairs. Indian J Surg. 2004;66:70-4.
10. Esposito C, Alicchio F, Giurin I, Castellano M, Settimi A. Technical standardization of laparoscopic direct hernia repair in pediatric patients. J Laparoendosc Adv Surg Tech A. 2012;22:113-6.
11. Nah SA, Giacomello L, Eaton S, de Coppi P, Curry JI, Drake DP, et al. Surgical repair of incarcerated inguinal hernia in children: laparoscopic or open? Eur J Pediatr Surg. 2011;21:8-11.

Chapter

16 Hybrid Hernia Repair

INTRODUCTION

Hernia is a very common disease that can be successfully managed through open surgery or laparoscopy. Laparoscopic surgery has clear advantages over open surgery such as lower morbidity (sepsis and pain), mortality, and shorter hospitalization. It has lesser risk of seroma, wound-related problems, and mesh-related problems. Multiple surgeries can be combined. Patients are more satisfied with returning to work earlier. A larger mesh can be placed in laparoscopy. In selected cases, open surgery outperformed laparoscopy. Larger defects, unsightly scars, aprons, and massive adhesions are few of them.

In some cases, open surgical steps were required along with laparoscopic steps. These cases account for 4.7% of the total hernia cases operated on by us. Other studies show an incidence of around 10%. This concept evolved into hybrid surgery, e.g., simultaneous open ventral hernia repair and total laparoscopic hysterectomy (TLH). Hybrid surgery in which laparoscopic and open surgical steps are applied to repair the hernia is called hybrid hernia repair.[1-3]

Hybrid surgery should not be an on-table decision or conversion to open due to difficulty or complication. That should be a preoperative decision.

TYPES

Hybrid hernia repair is classified based on open surgery done first or laparoscopy done first:

- *OL:* Open surgery and then laparoscopy
- *OLO:* Open surgery, then laparoscopy, which is followed by open surgery again
- *LO:* Laparoscopy followed by open surgery
- *LOL:* Laparoscopy followed by open surgery, then laparoscopy once more.

SANDWICH REPAIR

The abdominal wall is augmented on the outer and inner sides, with mesh on both sides or mesh on one side and a fascial flap on the other.[4]

TABLE 1: Open-favored adhesions and lap-favored adhesions.

	Open-favored adhesions	*Lap-favored adhesions*
Adhesion—site	Inside the sac of an irreducible hernia	Inside the abdominal cavity
Adhesion—content	Bowel/bladder incarcerated in scar tissue	Omentum
Adhesion—nature	Thick and fibrous	Thin
Need of the surgeon	Feel of tissue	Better vision and magnification

ADHESIONS (OPEN-FAVORED OR LAP-FAVORED) (TABLE 1)

Those adhesions where open surgery is better and safer than laparoscopy to perform adhesiolysis completely are known as open-favored adhesions.

Those adhesions where laparoscopy is preferred over open surgery due to access and visualization are known as lap-favored adhesions.

DEFECT PATTERN (OPEN-FAVORED OR LAP-FAVORED DEFECTS)

Like adhesions, defects are lap-favored or open-favored. Determinants of a defect pattern are: (1) Size of defect, (2) number of defects, and (3) nature of the surrounding muscles (divarication recti, paper-thin muscles,[5,6] muscle loss, and atrophy). In laparoscopy, a large mesh can be kept.[1] But larger defects requiring plication and darning (ventral defects >8 cm and inguinal defects >4 cm) are best closed through an open incision.[7] In incisional hernia after renal transplantation, some parts of the defect are better covered with a laparoscopically placed large mesh, while part of the defect overlying the transplanted kidney is better covered with an open onlay mesh.

In cases of bilateral inguinal hernia with a small umbilical defect <1 cm, the inguinal defects can be better managed laparoscopically. For umbilical hernia, being the primary trocar site, anatomical closure would be sufficient.

OL and OLO

In cases with multiple surgeries in the past, intra-abdominal adhesions, or an obstructed abdominal hernia, there is difficulty in placing the initial trocar because dense adhesions are expected at the laparoscopic entry site.[8,9] Open surgery and trocar placement under vision are safer in such cases.

Cases with a large skin apron, badly scarred skin, or the presence of multiple sinuses also required open surgery first. Trocars placed under the skin flap had excellent cosmesis and did not leave a scar on the exposed abdomen.

Apron: In cases of ventral hernia with a large apron, we raise the flap and place trocars. This avoided scarring in the umbilical and supraumbilical regions.

In patients with a history of enterocutaneous fistulas, three or more laparotomies, postoperative wound site infections, and mesh rejection, dense adhesions are to be expected. An incision is made to reduce the contents of the hernia, and trocars were placed under direct vision.

Presence of multiple sinuses: We remove the scar first because trocar placement could be planned based on skin lost and hernial defect. In cases of obstructed hernia, abdominal distention makes the initial trocar placement unsafe.

A skin incision is made that preserves enough healthy skin to get a cover and at the same time get a good cosmesis. The hernial sac is opened, adhesiolysis is performed, and the contents are reduced. Once the peritoneal cavity is reached, the primary trocar is placed under vision or under hand guidance. The hernial defect is closed with multiple Allis forceps or 1-0 polypropylene suture.

Then, laparoscopic working ports are placed, and laparoscopic surgery is performed. Laparoscopy helps to combine other surgeries. Adhesiolysis (lap-favored), placement of large mesh, and performing sandwich mesh repair are other advantages of laparoscopy. A mesh is placed laparoscopically in cases where open mesh placement is not possible due to long divarication, papery-thin muscles, and very little subcutaneous fat. Bridging gaps of muscle loss with laparoscopic mesh in cases with healed sinuses, scarring and colostomy reversal is better. Laparoscopy also helps to reduce the length of the open surgical incision.

After completion of laparoscopic procedures, final open steps are required in some cases. A mesh is placed for sandwich repair or darning is done from outside. In some cases with an apron, dermolipectomy is done and neoumbilicus is created. The skin incisions are then closed. These come under OLO **(Figs. 1 to 3)**.

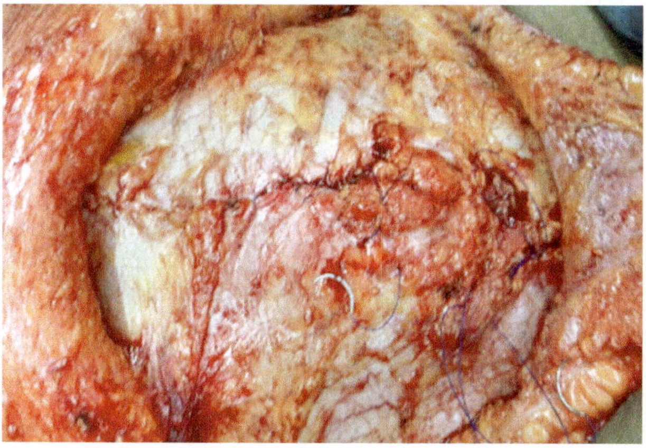

Fig. 1: Initial open surgery (OLO).

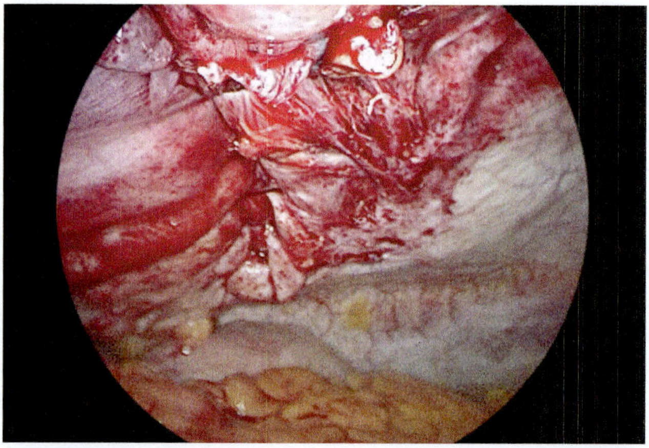

Fig. 2: Laparoscopic step (OLO).

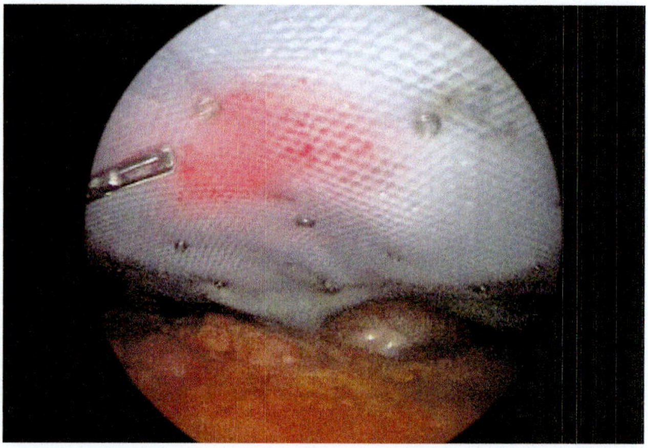

Fig. 3: Mesh placement laparoscopically (OLO).

LO and LOL

Initially, laparoscopic ports are placed. Dissection of the hernia is done laparoscopically as much as possible. After that, the skin above the hernia is cut **(Figs. 4 to 9)**.

The following steps are better done with open surgery:[1,2,5]

- Examination of contents
- Management of irreducibility and open-favored adhesions
- Removal of contents (omentum) and devitalized tissues
- Suturing or darning of the defect
- Sublay mesh repair
- Sandwich mesh repair, fascial flap, and component separation
- Removal of a large sac or scar to achieve better cosmesis.

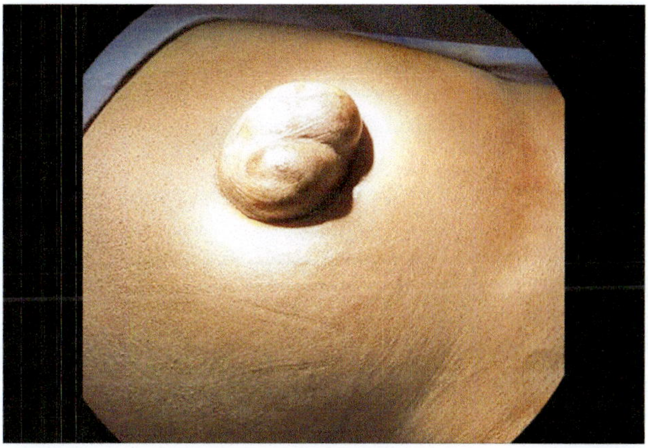

Fig. 4: Umbilical hernia (LO).

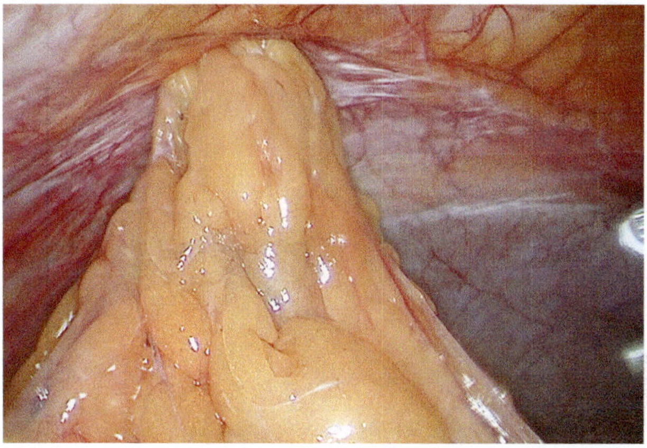

Fig. 5: Laparoscopic view (LO).

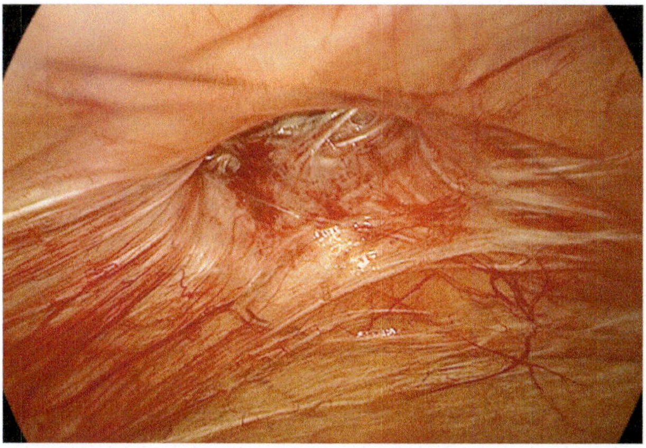

Fig. 6: Contents reduced (LO).

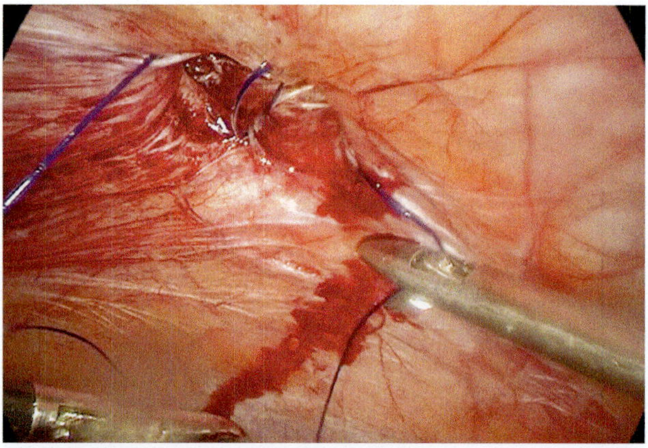

Fig. 7: Defect closure laparoscopically (LO).

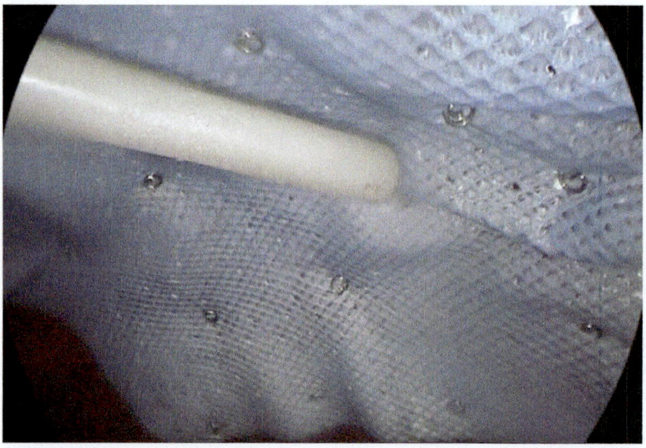

Fig. 8: Mesh placement laparoscopically (LO).

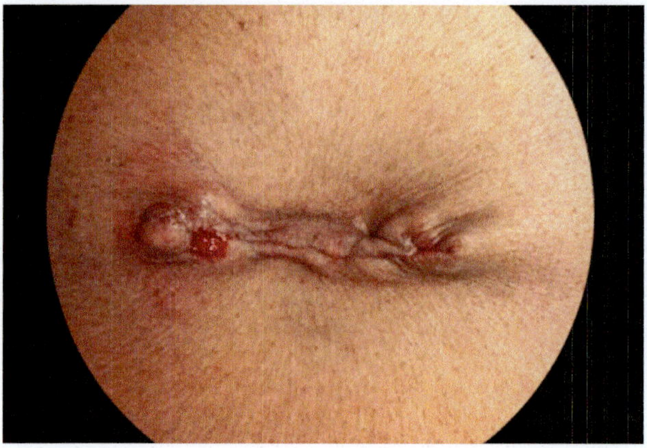

Fig. 9: Open surgery to remove the redundant sac (LO).

In some cases, laparoscopic mesh placement is performed after the open procedure. Those cases were classified by LOL **(Figs. 10 to 14)**.

Open mesh placement can be onlay, sublay, preperitoneal, or Lichtenstein with polypropylene meshes or partially absorbable meshes. Laparoscopic mesh placement can be preperitoneal, sublay [extended totally extraperitoneal (eTEP)] repair, or IPOM (intraperitoneal onlay mesh placement), using dual meshes or polypropylene meshes.

Hybrid surgery should be thought of in the following situations:[10-12]

- Ventral hernia with an apron and the need to combine other abdominal surgeries such as cholecystectomy, TLH, ovarian cystectomy, elective appendectomy, and sleeve gastrectomy—OLO

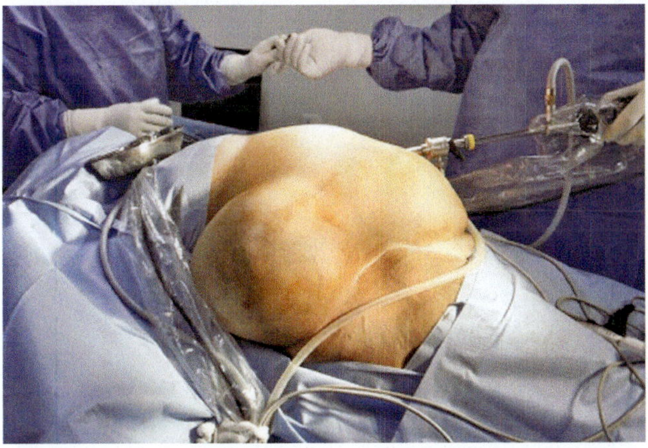

Fig. 10: Huge lumbar hernia (LOL).

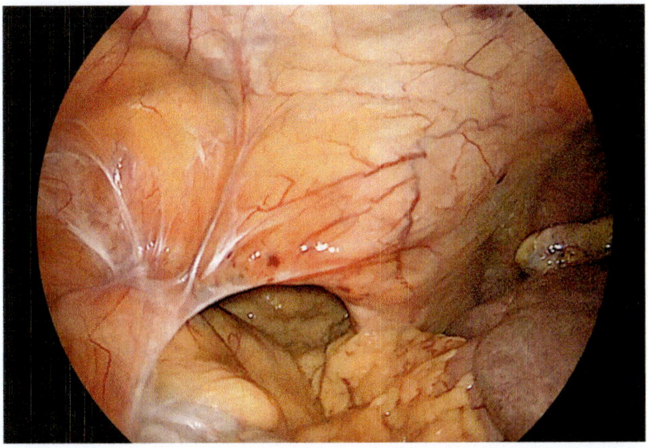

Fig. 11: Laparoscopic view of hernia (LOL).

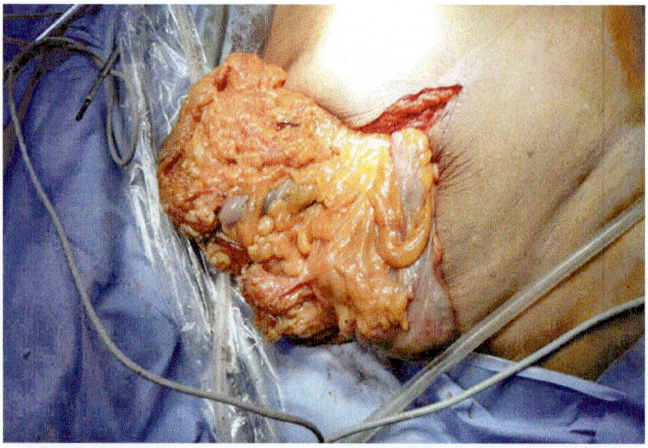

Fig. 12: Open surgery for correcting the hernia from outside (LOL).

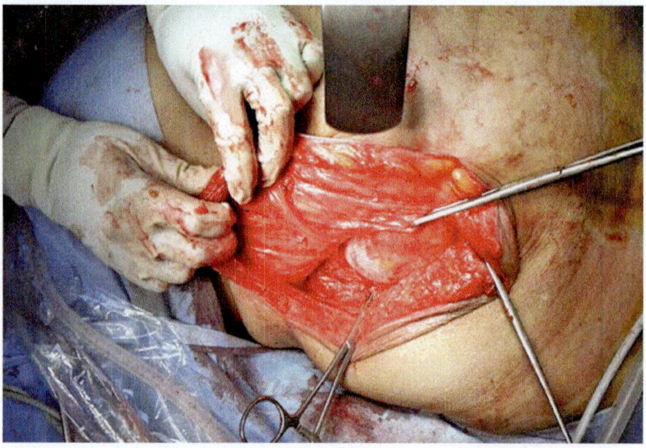

Fig. 13: Onlay mesh placement (LOL).

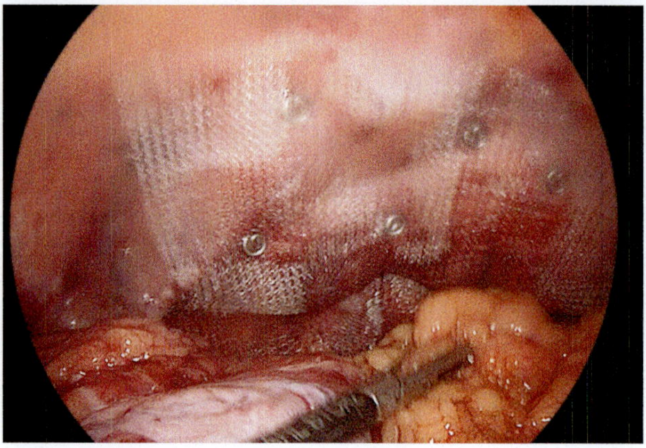

Fig. 14: Laparoscopic mesh placement (LOL).

- Ventral hernia without an apron, but irreducibility, need for omentectomy, and darning to close the defects—LO
- Inguinal hernia and the need for omentectomy—LOL
- Large defects (>8 cm in ventral hernia and >4 cm in inguinal hernia, relative), redundant sac, obesity, previous multiple abdominal surgeries, recurrent hernias, and presence of multiple precipitating factors are other factors favoring hybrid surgery.

Wasim et al. in their study compared laparoscopy and hybrid surgery.[9] Postoperative seroma, mesh protrusion, complicated adhesiolysis, and pain scores were lower in the hybrid group. Hybrid repair reduces recurrence rates.

TIPS AND TRICKS

An air leak occurred through the open incision. Multiple Allis forceps were used to approximate the defect to minimize this problem.

Lack of space occurs after abdominoplasty. When fascia is plicated, placing the mesh inside is difficult as the fascia hangs inside. If plication was performed after laparoscopic mesh placement, it led to mesh crumbling. It is necessary to anticipate difficulties and make a case-to-case adjustment.

In some cases, it is necessary to switch between laparoscopy and open surgery several times. Therefore, the closing of the walls is postponed until all other steps are completed. For the same reason, mesh placement is performed at the end of the procedure.

REFERENCES

1. Madhukara P, Padmakumar R, Premna S. Hybrid surgery in hernias: our experience. Kerala Surgical Journal. 2021;27(2):157-63.
2. Romanowska M, Pawlak J. Hybrid Technique for Incisional Hernias, Hernia Surgery and Recent Developments, Arshad M. Malik, IntechOpen, 2018; DOI: 10.5772/intechopen.76941. Available from: https://www.intechopen.com/chapters/61176.
3. Stoikes N, Quasebarth M, Brunt LM. Hybrid ventral hernia repair: technique and results. Hernia. 2013;17:627-32.
4. Köckerling F, Scheuerlein H, Schug-Pass C. Treatment of large incisional hernias in sandwich technique—A review of the literature. Front Surg. 2018;5:37.
5. Sauerland S, Walgenbach M, Habermalz B, Seiler CM, Miserez M. Laparoscopic versus open surgical techniques for ventral or incisional hernia repair. Cochrane Database Syst Rev. 2011;3:CD007781. [doi: 10.1002/14651858.CD007781.pub2].
6. Savitch SL, Shah PC. Closing the gap between the laparoscopic and open approaches to abdominal wall hernia repair: a trend and outcomes analysis of the ACS-NSQIP database. Surg Endosc. 2016;30:3267-78.
7. Kingsnorth A, Banerjea A, Bhargava A. Incisional hernia repair—Laparoscopic or open surgery? Ann R Coll Surg Engl. 2009;91:631-6. Available from: https://www.journalofmas.com/preprintarticle.asp?id=294953.

8. Sharma A, Sinha C, Baijal M, Soni V, Khullar R, Chowbey P. Hybrid approach for ventral incisional hernias of the abdominal wall: A systematic review of the literature. Min Access Surg 2021;17:7-13. Available from: https://www.journalofmas.com/preprintarticle.asp?id=294953. [Last accessed on 2020 Oct 27].
9. Wasim MD, Muddebihal UM, Rao UV. Hybrid: Evolving techniques in laparoscopic ventral hernia mesh repair. J Min Access Surg. 2020;16:224-8.
10. Meytes V, Lee A, Rivelis Y, Ferzli G, Timoney M. Hybrid fascial closure with laparoscopic mesh placement for ventral hernias: a single surgeon experience. Ann Laparosc Endosc Surg. 2017;2:55.
11. Shanker MC, Shanker K. Hybrid technique vs totally laparoscopic IPOM technique in ventral hernia—our experience. J Evol Med Dent Sci. 2018;7:5165-9.
12. Ahonen-Siirtola M, Nevala T, Vironen J, Kössi J, Pinta T, Niemeläinen S, et al. Laparoscopic versus hybrid approach for treatment of incisional ventral hernia: A prospective randomised multicentre study, 1-year results. Surg Endosc. 2020;34:88-95.

Chapter 17

Mesh and Mesh Fixatives

INTRODUCTION

A mesh is a barrier made of connected strands of metal, fiber, or other flexible or ductile materials. A mesh is similar to a web or a net in that it has many attached or woven strands.

Hernia is a weakness in the muscle and the protrusion of abdominal organs or part of organs (mostly the bowel or omentum) through muscle defect. Treatment of hernia was initially started by giving support from the outside like hernia belt or truss. Later, nonabsorbable sutures were used to repair the defect. These were replaced by woven meshes. The concept of mesh was first suggested by Theodore Billroth in 1890.[1] An ideal mesh was not found because most of the meshes that were produced failed due to infections and rejections. The father of the modern mesh is Francis Usher. In 1955, he used polyolefin material, i.e., Marlex mesh. In the 1980s, Lichtenstein came forward with a tension-free repair method and this is when the mesh was popularized. The mesh later found its way into laparoscopic surgeries.

WHY IS MESH USED?

When the defect is sutured, due to tension, the sutures may cut through and chances of recurrence of hernia are high. The concept of tension-free repair becomes possible only by using a mesh. It is less painful, stronger than the original tissue, and has a very low recurrence rate.

IDEAL MESH PROPERTIES[2]

- Chemically inert
- Incorporates rapidly into the host tissue
- Resistant to mechanical strain
- Flexible
- Ability to maintain long-term tensile strength to prevent a recurrence
- Resistant to infection
- Should not be carcinogenic
- Cost effective.

CLASSIFICATION OF MESH[3]

A mesh has got various characteristics, based on which it is classified.

- *Material of the mesh*
  - Biomaterial mesh
    - Alloderm—human derived
    - Surgisis—porcine derived
  - Synthetic mesh
    - Metallic mesh
    - Nonmetallic mesh
      - Polypropylene (monofilament)
      - Polyester (multifilament/braided)
      - Partially absorbable/composite mesh.

A polypropylene monofilamentous mesh is the most widely used mesh.

- *Weight of the mesh* **(Table 1)**

Commonly used are medium-weight meshes or lightweight meshes.

- *Porosity of mesh:*
  - Very large pores (>2 mm)
  - Large pores (macroporous) (1–2 mm)
  - Medium pore (0.6–1 mm)
  - Small pores (<0.6 mm)

Commonly used are medium—to large-pore meshes.

- *Design of meshes:*
  - Flat mesh
  - Dual-layer mesh
  - Anatomical
  - Self-gripping
  - Conical
- *Sizes available (in cm):*
  - 6 × 11
  - 10 × 15
  - 15 × 15

TABLE 1: Classification based on weight of the mesh.

Weight basis	*Weight*
Heavyweight	>140 g/m^2
Standard weight	70–140 g/m^2
Medium weight	50–70 g/m^2
Lightweight	35–50 g/m^2
Ultra lightweight	<35 g/m^2

- 12 × 18
- 10 × 20
- 30 × 30

▪ *Classification based on the textile structure of the fibers of mesh* **(Table 2)**
  - *Raw materials and mesh composition:*
    - Nonabsorbable materials—polypropylene, polyethylene terephthalate (PET), expanded polytetrafluoroethylene (ePTFE)
    - Absorbable materials—polylactic acid (PLA), polyglycolic acid (PGA).

Polypropylene meshes result in an intensified inflammatory reaction. More collagen fibers are deposited and there are significantly higher

TABLE 2: Types of mesh fabrics.[4]

Textile structure		*Definition*
Knitted fabric	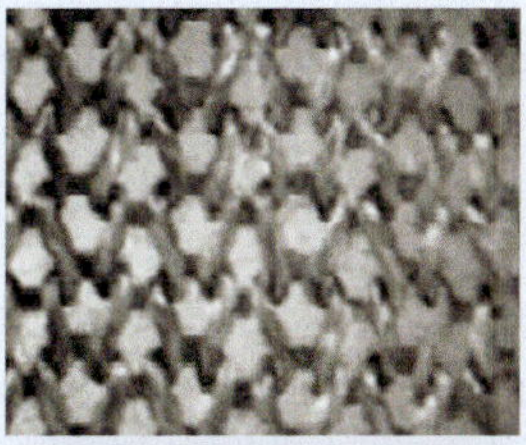	Knitted fabric consists of a single thread that forms a number of consecutive rows of loops. Trimming of knitted structures often leads to a complete failure of the mesh
Warp-knitted fabric	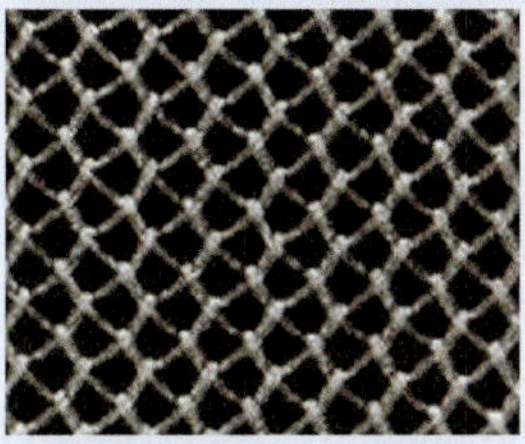	Warp-knitted fabric consists of multiple threads forming loops. In contrast to knitted structures, warp-knitted structures can be trimmed and sewed
Nonwoven fabric	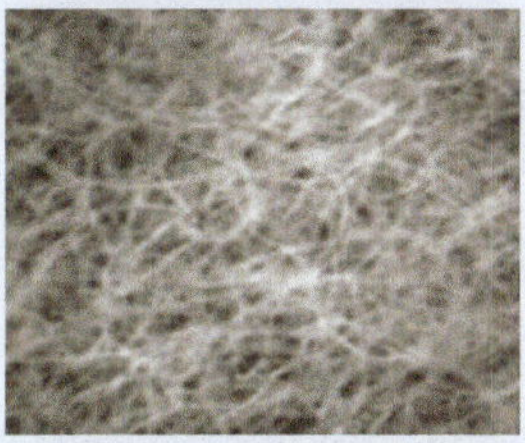	Nonwoven fabric consists of nonorientated or to a certain degree orientated, endless fibers. After the nonwoven formation the structure needs to be bonded by either mechanical, thermal, or chemical bonding
Woven fabric	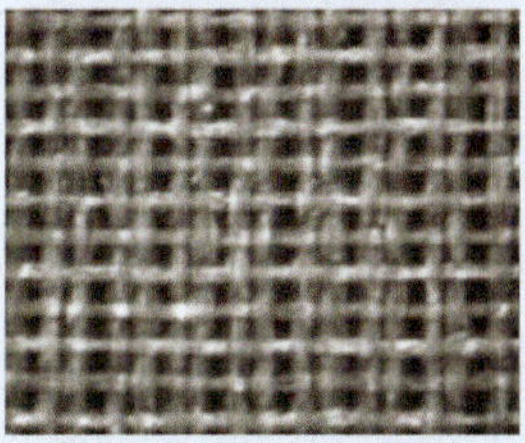	Woven structures consist of two distinct sets of yarns or threads which are interlaced at right angles to form a fabric

collagen type I/III ratios. The resulting scar tissue is stronger compared with ePTFE meshes. So, a polypropylene mesh is more widely used.

WHAT HAPPENS WHEN WE KEEP THE MESH—THE INFLAMMATORY PROCESS[5]

The inflammatory process has four stages:

1. *Stage I*—coagulum formation
2. *Stage II*—acute inflammatory response (neutrophil migration) which gets converted to chronic inflammatory response
3. *Stage III*—chronic inflammation. Macrophages fuse into a foreign body giant cell formation and fibrotic response
4. *Stage IV*—collagen deposition and scar formation.

Cell migration is followed by collagen deposition. Initially, type 1 collagen is deposited, which in time gets converted into type 3 collagen.

The majority of tissue ingrowth and strength may be completed 2 weeks after mesh implantation, but the final remodeling happens over a long period of time.

By the end of 3 months, the inflammation decreases as these cells are replaced by healthy connective tissue (or scar tissue).

Intense or prolonged inflammation, bad infiltration, and immature collagen deposition result in unhealthy scar plate formation, which can be accompanied by increased stiffness of the abdominal wall, shrinkage or deformation of the biomaterial leading to recurrence, adhesion, fistula, or erosion of nearby tissue.

MESH PROPERTIES

Mesh Weight—Pore Size

Usually, when the pore size increases, the material in the mesh is reduced, so the mesh becomes lighter; lightweight meshes are usually macroporous, while heavy meshes are microporous. In a macroporous mesh, the fibrosis happens at the periphery of each pore and the central part remains flexible so the cross bridging of the fibrosed tissue does not happen. The chances of mesh shrinkage will be less, and the scar plate will be more flexible, and a less stiff scar plate reduces pain. If the mesh is very macroporous, the material in the mesh will be lesser and the strength of the mesh reduces. The chances of rupture of the mesh and recurrence happen. Also, when we fix with tackers, when the pore is very large the tacks would not hold and the mesh may fall off.

Mesh Memory

Memory is the ability of a mesh to return to its original shape after introduction into the surgical field. It varies between meshes; some lightweight microporous mesh has no memory, so they remain crumbled. Memory is a mechanical parameter that is important for handling the mesh during deployment. Usually, meshes with good memory are preferred for laparoscopy.

Mesh Shrinkage

Most meshes shrink up to 60% of their original size. A larger mesh with 5 cm overlap from the margin of the defect of hernia is preferred.

COMMONLY USED MESHES AND THEIR PROPERTIES

Monofilament Polypropylene (Fig. 1)

- Pores (2.0 × 2.4 mm)
- Wrap knitting construct—provides easy mesh handling, abdominal wall conformability, and can be trimmed to size without fraying.
- It has a surface density of 46 g/m^2.
- Transparent—improved visualization to aid mesh placement and fixation.
- Memory shape—the right balance between rigidity and softness.

Dual Mesh

The dual-layer mesh has two layers **(Fig. 2)**:

1. Polypropylene which goes to the abdominal wall
2. Antiadhesive layer facing the intestines, which prevents the adhesion of the bowel

Theoretical studies do favor dual-layered mesh over normal polypropene, but there are an equal number of studies which favor the regular polypropylene mesh for intraperitoneal placement with similar or no added complications.

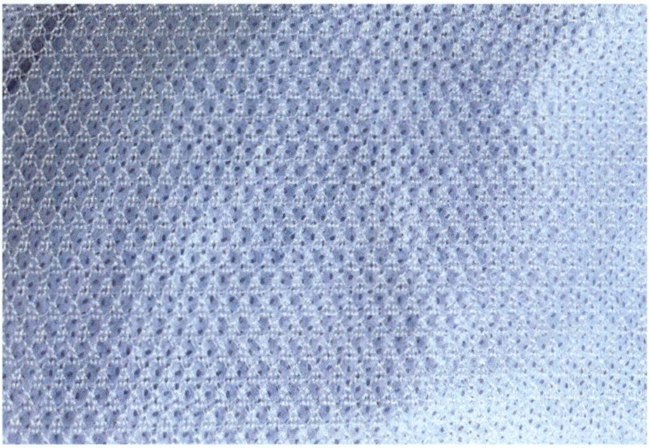

Fig. 1: Polypropylene.

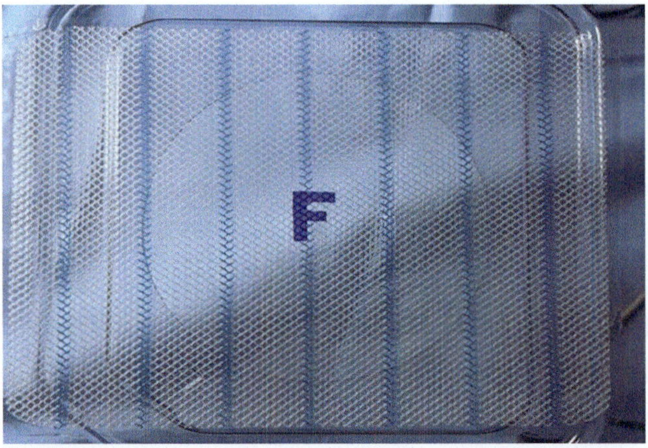

Fig. 2: Dual mesh. F shows the center and nonadhesive side.

NEWER TYPES OF MESHES

- 3D meshes*
- Self-gripping meshes*
- Antibiotic impregnated meshes (ampicillin, gentamicin, cefazolin, vancomycin, levofloxacin + silver)
    - *Titanium-coated meshes:* These have a nonadhesive property irrespective of the side facing the bowel.

Note: When doing an open hernia repair, we can apply gentamicin over the mesh after fixation to prevent an infection.

COMPLICATIONS OF MESH

Seroma Formation

Seroma formation is the most common complication that may arise (20% of the cases show swelling in the hernial sac). It resolves with time. Conservative management is the preferred treatment of choice. Seroma can be prevented by inverting and obliterating the sac with tacks or with external pressure dressings.

Hematoma

Hematoma may be due to bleeding from the dissected surface or due to vascular injury (inferior epigastric vessels/retropubic veins). Care must be given to prevent bleeding and early control once it happens. It leads to mesh displacement, infection, and recurrence of hernia.

*Claims ease of application but is an expensive option.

Infection

Mesh is a foreign body and if a hematoma is formed around the mesh, there is a chance that the mesh gets displaced and may become infected.

Ways to prevent mesh infection are as follows:

- Gentle dissection and prevention of hematoma
- Administer prophylactic antibiotics at the time of induction. If the surgery time is prolonged for >3 hours, a second dose of antibiotics has to be administered.
- Before handling the mesh, the surgeon must change gloves. The mesh must be given directly to the surgeon. If the mesh needs to be cut, a separate sterile scissors must be used. The mesh should not come in contact with the skin of the patient or on to the trolley. It must be directly folded and put to the abdomen of the patient. If multiple meshes are to be placed, then gloves must be changed before handling each mesh.

In case of mesh infection, patients will be toxic with fever as well as pain and swelling at the hernia site. On ultrasound examination, it may be difficult to differentiate between hematoma and infection. Needle aspiration may yield seropurulent or purulent material, which can be sent for culture and sensitivity.

When a mesh infection is suspected, the initial treatment can be a course of broad-spectrum antibiotics. If a culture is done, then culture-based antibiotics may be given. Antitubercular treatment can be tried after an antibiotic course if there is no improvement.

If infection is not getting controlled after conservative management, the mesh may be removed by either laparoscopy or open surgery.

Adhesions

As a mesh causes fibrotic response, bowel or omentum close to the mesh can get adhered to the mesh and may lead to intestinal obstruction. Rarely, the mesh erodes the bowel and leads to fistula formation.

Recurrence of Hernia after Mesh Plasty

Causes:

- Shrinkage of mesh
- Weakening of the abdominal wall
- When the defect is not sutured, the entire mesh can cup into the defect and cause cupping of the mesh.
- Hematoma/seroma displacing the mesh
- Mesh removal due to infection
- Smaller mesh than required
- Faulty technique—improper placement of mesh
- Inadequate dissection.

Postoperative Pain

Prolonged pain usually happens due to mesh fixatives and also the nerve entrapment into the fibrous tissue of the mesh. It usually resolves in a few months' time with analgesics or pregabalin. If the pain is severe, local anesthetics and steroids can be given under ultrasound guidance at the point of maximum pain.

The surgeon has to be careful while applying tacks and make sure to avoid areas such as the trapezoid, close proximity of epigastric vessels, and pelvic bone. Too tight tissue approximation by sutures is also to be avoided to prevent tissue ischemia and resultant pain. Good analgesics in the initial postoperative days will break the pain cycle and avoid chronic pain.

MESH FIXATIVES

Primary function of a fixation device is to keep the mesh in its position until the mesh gets incorporated into the abdominal wall. In open surgeries, sutures are used. In laparoscopy, suturing is a time-consuming procedure; hence, better devices such as tacks are used. Tack is the pin which is used to fix the mesh. The instrument used to deliver the tack is called a tacker. Tacks can be metallic or absorbable. Metallic, i.e., titanium-based, tacks are used more often. Tissue glues and staples are also used to fix the mesh.[6]

In the case of totally extraperitoneal repair, it is said that fixation is not necessary but we fix the mesh at least at two points.

HELICAL TITANIUM TACKS

Helical titanium tack has a helical shape, measures 4 mm in length and 3 mm in width, and penetrates approximately 3–4 mm into fascia and muscle of

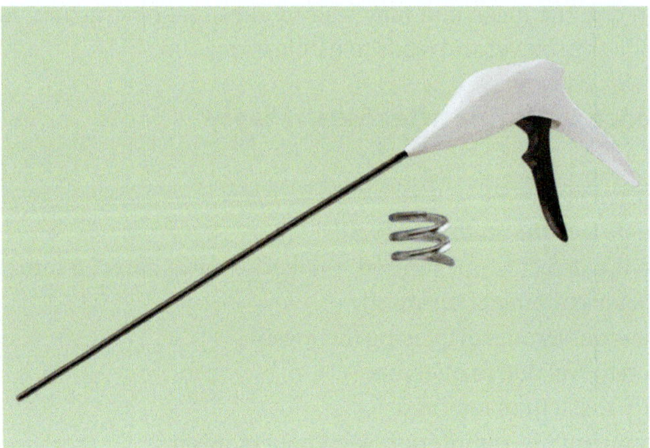

Fig. 3: Nonabsorbable tacker.

the anterior abdominal wall. For ventral hernia, tacks must be placed 3–4 cm apart, along the periphery of the mesh to avoid folding of mesh. Another round of tacks is applied around the hernia defect **(Fig. 3)**.

ABSORBABLE TACKERS

Penetration of the absorbable tack is less deep and it is difficult to sterilize by ethylene oxide sterilization (ETO). For these reasons, absorbable tackers are less popular.

DOS WHEN WE TACK

Counterpressure must be applied from outside to make the tissue perpendicular to the tacker and must be closely approximated.

The gun should be fired to its full extent without hesitation and then released.

DON'TS FOR MESH AND TACKS

- Reuse of mesh
- Reuse of tackers without ETO
- Not changing gloves before handling the mesh
- Cutting and trimming of dual-layer mesh
- Using mesh in the presence of infection
- Insufficient size of mesh
- Ultra lightweight mesh.

INGUINAL MESH FIXATION

Place one tack at the suprapubic region, one tack just below umbilicus in the midline, and one tack laterally. If the mesh is getting lifted, then a tack is put on Cooper's ligament **(Fig. 4)**.

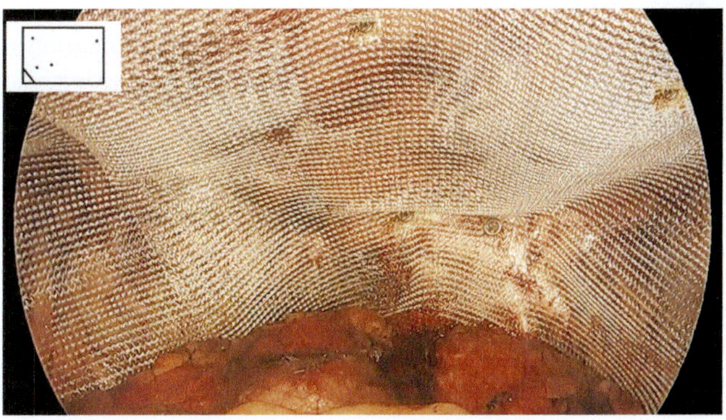

Fig. 4: Fixing of the inguinal mesh.

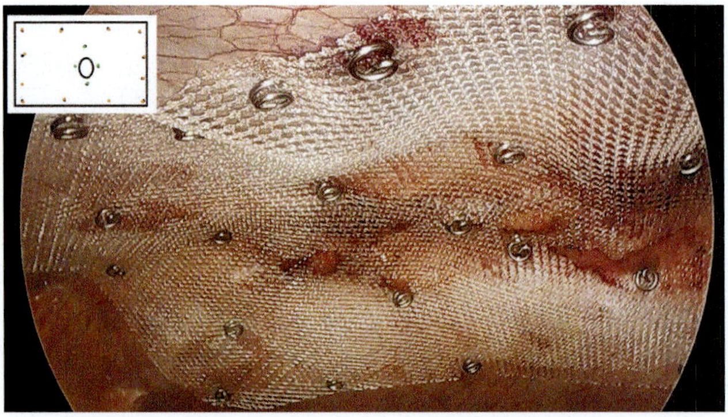

Fig. 5: Double crowning of mesh in ventral hernia.

VENTRAL MESH FIXATION

In ventral hernia, use a double-crown technique i.e., 4 tacks around the defect and 9–12 tacks at the periphery of the mesh **(Fig. 5)**. The inner crown prevents falling of the mesh from the abdominal wall. The outer crown maintains mesh alignment and prevents bowel coming in between the mesh and the abdominal wall. This technique helps in reducing recurrence.

REFERENCES

1. Hee RV. History of inguinal hernia repair. Jurnalul de Chirurgie, Iaşi. 2011;7(3).
2. Bringman S, Conze J, Cuccurullo D, Deprest J, Junge K, Klosterhalfen B, et al. Hernia repair: the search for ideal meshes. Hernia. 2010;14(1):81-7.
3. Klinge U, Klosterhalfen B. Modified classification of surgical meshes for hernia repair based on the analyses of 1,000 explanted meshes. Hernia. 2012;16(3):251-8.
4. Zhu LM, Schuster P, Klinge U. Mesh implants: an overview of crucial mesh parameters. World J Gastrointest Surg 2015; 7(10): 226-36.
5. Baylón K, Rodríguez-Camarillo P, Elías-Zúñiga A, Díaz-Elizondo JA, Gilkerson R, Lozano K. Past, Present and Future of Surgical Meshes: A Review. Membranes (Basel). 2017;7(3):47.
6. Mathes T, Prediger B, Walgenbach M, Siegel R. Mesh fixation techniques in primary ventral or incisional hernia repair. Cochrane Database Syst Rev. 2021;5(5).

Chapter

18 Difficulties and Complications: How to Troubleshoot?

INTRODUCTION

Hernia repair has evolved over more than 150 years. Various procedures have been advocated, and each has its own merits and demerits. When done with due care and knowledge, each procedure has good results and the same applies to laparoscopy also, the key to success being:

- Thorough knowledge of anatomy
- Training under a good surgeon—someone should make you do it.
- Due care given to assessing the patient during the preoperative, intraoperative, postoperative, and follow-up visits. The same tempo should be kept from beginning to end. You may fail at any level, so each step is important.
- Gentle handling of tissues and patients. Gentle dissection is vital to any surgery. If you handle tissues badly, they will react badly. Similarly, due care should be provided for a patient's concerns and quality of life.

Although laparoscopy aims at reducing difficulties during surgery and also morbidity induced by the procedure, a new set of problems as well as some of the old ones are being experienced. This chapter aims at describing these difficulties encountered during surgery and complications thereafter and their management to the present-day knowledge.

DIFFICULTIES ENCOUNTERED DURING LAPAROSCOPIC HERNIA REPAIR

The difficulties that arise during laparoscopic hernia repair can be grouped under two heads, those possible in open surgical procedures as well and those specific to laparoscopic hernia repair. The first group includes bleeding and difficulty arising in the form of irreducibility and strangulation, while the second group involves anatomy-related and technique-related issues.

Hemorrhage

During laparoscopic hernia repair, bleeding can occur from three different zones. It can occur from:

1. Inferior epigastric vessels
2. External iliac vessels
3. Deep venous plexus of pelvis.

Inferior epigastric vessels can bleed during trocar placement, peritoneal dissection, or application of tack **(Fig. 1)**. It can be avoided by placing 5 mm trocars lateral to the rectus sheath and also identification of the vessels prior to lateral dissection. Once it occurs, it can be controlled by pressure with an instrument and coagulated with a sealing device such as a bipolar/harmonic scalpel or clipped on the cut ends.

Another case of troublesome bleed is from external iliac vessels which can even be life threatening due to loss of blood or even an air embolism. It should be controlled immediately with pressure. If it is not possible to tackle by laparoscopic means, we can convert to open immediately and tackle the bleeder. We should give due respect to the iliac vessels and be very gentle in handling these structures and once again, a thorough knowledge of anatomy is most needed.

Bleeding can occur from the deep venous plexus of pelvis, and these vessels bleed continuously in the loose potential space **(Fig. 2)**. The vision gets darkened and dissection becomes difficult. Avoid rough handling of background tissues and if bleeding occurs, do not panic. Give a good wash, identify the bleeder, and control it with an energy source.

If there is bleeding, it is better to take care of bleeding before placing the mesh. The field becomes very dark with blood and it becomes difficult for the surgeon to operate. Use of suction irrigation makes the field clear but leads to a lot of wetness of tissues. A gauze piece inserted inside is preferred for wiping and taking care of the bleeding as it gives a dry field. Drain is usually not preferred because it can be a site of infection.

Irreducible or Strangulated Hernia

Usually with muscle relaxation and pneumoperitoneum, the bowel gets reduced **(Fig. 3)**. At times, it will be incarcerated. Dissect gently with a

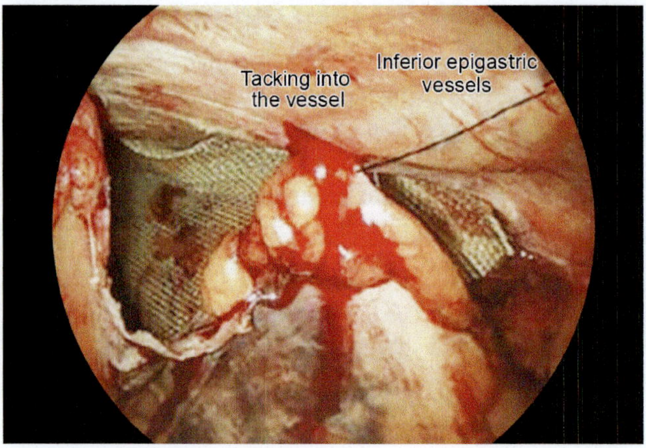

Fig. 1: Inferior epigastric artery caught in tack.

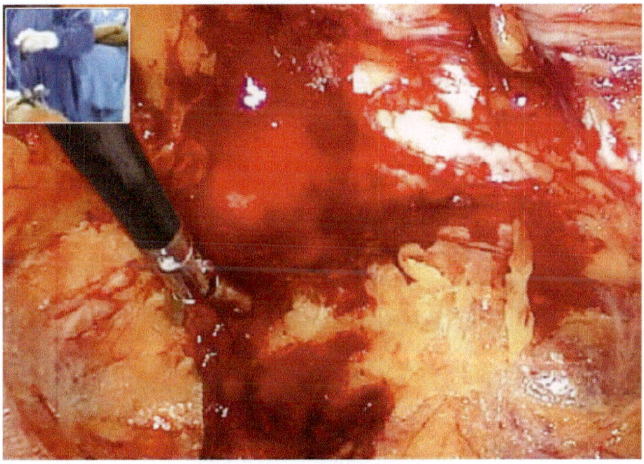

Fig. 2: Pelvic vessel bleeding.

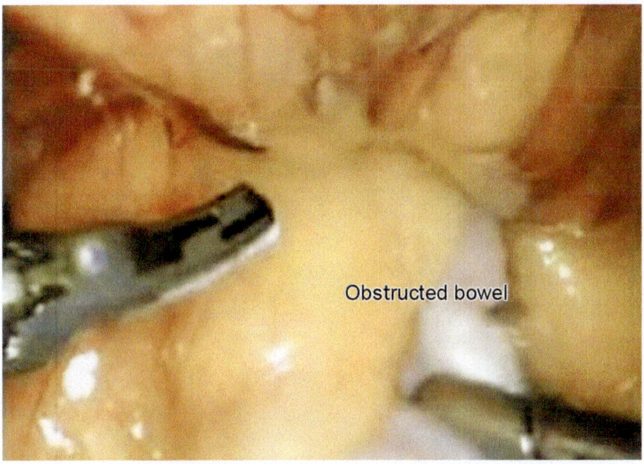

Fig. 3: Reduction of obstructed bowel.

bowel-holding forceps and a bipolar/harmonic scalpel to divide adhesions. The bowel can be reduced most often.

Rarely, in indirect sacs with a tight neck, a lateral incision can be made at the neck or else a small incision can be made over the inguinal region to admit the index finger to dilate the neck and reduce the contents.

If the content is the omentum, omentectomy can be done and the contents removed through an inguinal incision. In case the bowel is being strangulated, the plan to proceed with the mesh repair depends on the vascularity of the bowel and the inflammation of the hernial sac **(Figs. 4 and 5)**.

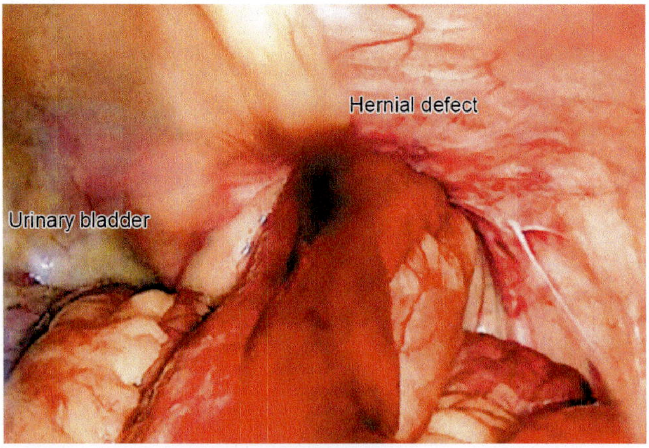

Fig. 4: Strangulated bowel.

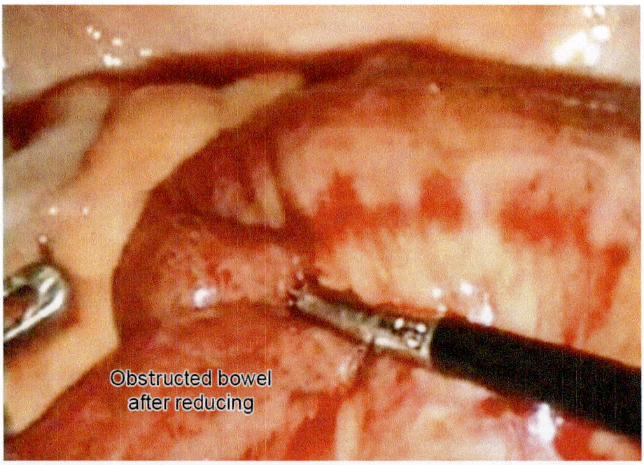

Fig. 5: Bowel regaining its color.

Problems Related to Different Anatomy

The major problem faced by most of the surgeons who try learning lap hernia repair is difficulty in understanding anatomy by the posterior approach. It becomes difficult to identify structures and even to see the hernial sac. At times, a hernial sac may be overlooked, which will lead to immediate postoperative recurrence. It is still difficult in situations where the iliac vessels, nerves, bowel, or even the bladder gets injured during the procedure. A thorough knowledge of posterior approach anatomy is a must before attempting laparoscopic hernia repair. It can be obtained from textbooks, 3D models, through open preperitoneal mesh repair/Stoppa repair for inguinal hernia, through a sublay repair for ventral hernia, through surgical videos by eminent surgeons, and, finally, by assisting a good surgeon who gives hands-on training.

At times it may be difficult even for experienced surgeons to decipher anatomy as in the case of recurrent hernias or those with intraperitoneal adhesions. Anatomy may not be clear or even may be altered. In such situations, decisions may be taken as per the expertise available. In your initial learning curve you may proceed with an open procedure, but experienced surgeons stick to the laparoscopic approach. They start their dissection far laterally in an uninvolved region and gradually dissect the preperitoneum and complete the procedure rather than dissecting into the adhesions.

Problems Related to Laparoscopic Technique

Few difficulties can arise during laparoscopic hernia repair, which are related to the technique per se. These include lack of working space, crowding of trocars, difficulties in dissection, etc. Lack of working space can occur due to air leak at: (1) The trocar level with valve/washer problems, (2) larger skin incisions, or (3) leak occurring in the peritoneum in totally extraperitoneal (TEP) repair. If the leak is outside, change of washer or trocar or keeping gauze will help. If it is due to peritoneal tear, you should keep yourself calm and continue the dissection. If it is not possible, convert to transabdominal preperitoneal (TAPP) repair, and the problem will be solved. Check for liquid gas volume of the cylinder, pressure kept at insufflator being 12–15 mm Hg and also whether adequate relaxation is given.

Proper placement of working ports is a requirement for any laparoscopic procedure. In TEP repair, trocars can get crowded and hit each other. Putting lateral trocars after dissection will help in dissecting the hernia better. In case of ventral hernia repair, instruments can hit the thigh of the patient or chest wall. Trocars may be changed as per your requirements or additional trocar put. This knowledge is usually gained through experience.

Usually, preperitoneal space dissects easily. But at times, the tissues will be more fibrotic and dissection will be difficult. In that scenario, continue with slow and careful dissection and try to understand every structure clearly before it is divided.

COMPLICATIONS

General Anesthesia-related Complications

These complications can occur with any of the procedures. Urinary retention can occur and the patient may require catheterization, especially in the elderly. Ileus can occur as with any other abdominal surgery. The explanations of these are beyond the scope of this book.

Complications of Laparoscopic Hernia Repair

Bowel Injury

Bowel injury can occur during trocar insertion or dissection. Care during the insertion of primary trocar, inspecting the site of entry before positioning the patient, and gentle and careful dissection will prevent this complication. If detected intraoperatively, suture closing the injury may be the way out; however, continuing with hernia repair may not be advisable if gross contamination has occurred. Situations become more difficult where injury is detected in postoperative period with feculent peritonitis. Re-exploration and stabilization of the patient will be advisable in this scenario **(Fig. 6)**.

Intestinal Obstruction

Intestinal obstruction may happen in cases of TAPP repair and rarely in cases of TEP repair where peritoneal rent leads to exposure of mesh and bowel adhesion. At times, the bowel can get adhered to the tack. Rarely, the bowel can herniate at the site of closure of peritoneum. The time of presentation may vary from the immediate postoperative period to even years after the procedure. It can be minimized by closing the site of peritoneal dissection properly and minimizing the occurrence of rents. The rents can be closed/covered with the omentum so as to minimize the exposure to bowel. In case of intraperitoneal mesh repair, the mesh should be properly fixed. Usage of dual mesh and covering with omentum during desufflation reduce the chance of bowel adhesions.

Seromas and Hematomas

Usually, seromas and hematomas occur in 2–10% of cases of laparoscopic hernia repair. They should be differentiated from a recurrence of hernia by

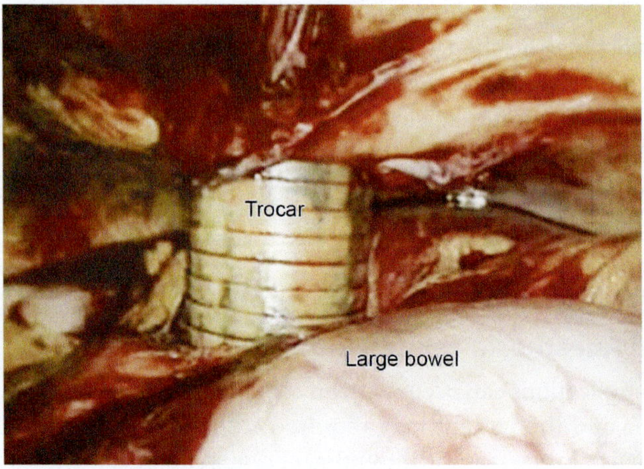

Fig. 6: Trocar injury.

careful clinical examination and sonological guidance. They usually resolve if left as such. Occasionally, they may require aspiration which needs to be repeated in only very few patients. Obliteration of sac with sutures/tacks reduces the incidence of seroma formation as is the use of pressure dressings. Rarely, a distal indirect sac may persist as hydrocele. In this case, it may be tackled with eversion of the sac later.

Cord Structure Injury

Injury to vas deferens and spermatic cord vessels are not so common after laparoscopic repair. Ischemic orchitis occurs in 3–5% cases of open repair but is rare in laparoscopy. It is because of better vision and gentle handling of tissues and avoidance of dissection of cord in case of huge indirect hernias. In laparoscopy, a mesh does not encircle the cord. In case of recurrent hernias and huge indirect hernias, spermatic cord and vessels are to be identified before dissecting any longitudinal structure lateral to the inferior epigastric vessels. Chronic orchialgia can occur after hernia repair, which is difficult to respond to analgesics. Addition of amitriptyline or gabapentin may be of help to those patients.

Mesh-related Complications

Mesh infection and rejection are accepted complications of mesh repair irrespective of the open/laparoscopic technique. These can be reduced by lowering the exposure of mesh to surroundings, i.e., open the mesh at the time of introduction, change your gloves while holding the mesh, use clean instruments to handle the mesh, and avoid hematoma formation with gentle dissection. Preoperative antibiotics reduce the chances of surgical site infection. Genta impregnation may be done to reduce the chance of infection, especially when it is sublay mesh repair.

If it occurs, pus can be aspirated and culture and sensitivity done, and antibiotics are started based on the sensitivity pattern. Even in the absence of infection, individuals can develop rejection of the mesh. Antitubercular treatment may be given a trial. If it does not respond, the mesh needs to be removed, which may be accomplished by the laparoscopic method as the mesh is located in a deeper plane.

Chronic Pain

Chronic pain can occur if any nerve gets entangled in the tack. The patient can continue analgesics, amitriptyline, and gabapentin. If the ultrasound scan shows tack at the site of the pain, injections of local anesthetic or removal of tack may relieve the patient of pain.

Chapter 19

Frequent Queries and Answers from Experts

1. **Case selection—Open surgery or laparoscopy**

   Laparoscopy: It can be done in almost all cases unless the patient is too fragile to tolerate anesthesia. For strangulated gangrenous bowel inside the sac, which is not getting reduced, laparoscopy may be difficult. Recurrent hernias, irreducible and early strangulated hernias, and rare hernias like lumbar are better tackled laparoscopically by experienced hands.

2. **Anesthesia—general anesthesia (GA)/spinal anesthesia**

   General anesthesia.

   Totally extraperitoneal (TEP) repair can be done under spinal or epidural analgesia, but gas leak/conversions to transabdominal preperitoneal (TAPP) repair may be a problem. This can be attempted in those patients who are not fit for general anesthesia. But in them, open repair under local analgesia and sedation may be the best option.

3. **Catheterization and Ryle's tube (RT) aspiration**

   Ryle's tube aspiration—no (except to decompress the stomach, which is palpably distended during anesthesia)

   Catheterization—rarely needed.

   The patient is made to pass urine immediately before being taken to the operation theater. Catheterization is needed in recurrent cases, obstructed hernias (bladder may be adherent or involved), and those with severe prostatism. For the last group, transurethral resection of prostate (TURP) in combination will be a better option. Otherwise, discontinuation of the catheter use may be difficult in the postoperative period.

4. **Approach—TEP/TAPP Repair**

   Totally extraperitoneal:

   - Tall, thin individuals; good distance between umbilicus and pubic symphysis
   - Direct/small indirect hernias which are reducible
   - Should be avoided in recurrent hernias or in irreducible hernias

- Should be avoided in right inguinal hernia after open appendicectomy and inguinofemoral hernias in postcesarean female patients—as preperitoneum will not get dissected
- Similar is the case to any other previous lower abdominal procedures

Transabdominal preperitoneal repair:

- Preferred where multiple procedures are to be combined, i.e., hernia and cholecystectomy, hernia and total laparoscopic hysterectomy, and small umbilical defect with inguinal hernia
- In irreducible/strangulated hernias
- Helps to inspect and tackle the opposite side while doing unilateral hernia repair.

5. **Use of energy source**

   Use of energy source is to be reduced to minimum. Dissection is done with scissors, Maryland forceps, monopolar hook, or harmonic scalpel. Combined sharp and blunt dissection needs to be done, and coagulation is used for vessels only. While using an energy source, especially in TEP repair, one should be careful about the bowel near the other side of the thin peritoneum.

6. **Prophylactic repair of opposite side**

   When doing TAPP repair for hernia repair on one side, and during surgery, if bubonocele is found in the opposite side, then bilateral repair is done. While doing TEP repair, the opposite side is not dissected to check the presence of hernia. So, if you are suspicious of the opposite side hernia, TAPP repair may be advisable.

   Some do advocate bilateral mesh repair for unilateral direct hernia in elderly as the patient has a higher chance of developing opposite side hernia, and relaparoscopy at that time will be difficult.

7. **Indirect sac excision/reduction**

   If the sac is small, it can be reduced, but if it is large, dissection of the sac leads to an increased chance of hematoma and seroma formation and ischemic orchitis. So, traction is applied and the sac is transected as distal as possible.

   In TEP repair, before transection of sac, maximum dissection is completed, otherwise leak of air into peritoneum can lead to loss of space and difficulty in dissection. Another option is ligation of the neck of sac before division.

8. **Type of mesh for extraperitoneal use**

   The usual polypropylene mesh is used. A lightweight mesh is not preferred as the placement will be difficult.

For intraperitoneal mesh placement, when the peritoneal cover is not possible, a dual mesh is preferred by some surgeons as the chances of adhesion are proposed to be lesser compared to the polypropylene mesh. However, we generally use a polypropylene mesh unless the patient is keen on having a dual mesh.

Extended TEP (eTEP)/transversus abdominis release (TAR) is preferred by some surgeons to circumvent the issue of having polypropylene mesh intraperitoneally.

9. **Need of TAR/hybrid**

   Hernias with very large defects may necessitate hybrid or TAR techniques of hernioplasty.

10. **Closure of peritoneal defect**

    Peritoneal defect may be closed to prevent herniation of bowel/ adhesion to the exposed posterior aspect of the mesh. It can be done with sutures/tacks. During desufflation, omentum can be used to cover the bowel to prevent bowel adhesion.

11. **Seroma prevention**

    Gentle dissection and avoidance of oozing will definitely reduce the chance of postoperative hematoma/seroma formation. In case of huge direct sacs, a pseudosac may be inverted and tacked medially to prevent seroma. This will also form a base on which the mesh will stay. Indirect sac, if huge, should not be dissected but divided as distal as possible. Keeping a pressure pad in the postoperative period for a day and then wearing tight undergarments or abdominal binder for ventral hernia will reduce the seroma formation.

    Seroma is seen as a swelling in the postoperative period, and it usually simulates an immediate recurrence of hernia. On careful palpation, cough impulse, even if present, will be slight. A cystic swelling will be felt moving over the abdominal muscles.

    Diagnosis can be confirmed with ultrasound examinations; if needed—may be aspirated to dryness. It subsides by itself, but occasionally requires repeated aspirations.

12. **Mesh infection prevention**

    - Preoperative antibiotics
    - Open the mesh just before its placement
    - Change the gloves
    - Clean trocar and instruments before holding the mesh
    - Good hemostasis
    - Proper sterilization of instruments and operation theater asepsis.

13. **Strangulated hernia**

Usually with muscle relaxation of general anesthesia, bowel will get reduced spontaneously. If strangulation is suspected, do not reduce the hernia before trocar placement as you will lose the chance to inspect the bowel inside it.

Once the bowel is seen stuck inside, it is reduced gently with bowel-holding forceps. Check for the vascularity of the bowel and also the condition of the hernial sac and the abdominal wall. If vascularity of bowel is regained, it could be left as such and mesh repair of hernia is done. If the bowel is devascularized, resection and anastomosis are done by taking out the bowel by enlarging the umbilical incision. In such a case, and also when the abdominal wall shows severe inflammation, mesh repair is deferred to a later date, preferably 6 weeks later. One may use biomesh in this situation.

14. **Rest and activity**

- Ambulate on the day of the surgery after 4 hours once the effect of sedation is over.
- After 24 hours of surgery, the patient is allowed to walk regularly, without any effort on the abdomen. Climbing stairs and light activity can be started 1 day after
- After discharge, passive sex may be permissible.
- In a week's time, all the works and active sexual contact can be started.
- Treadmill—3 weeks
- All activities may be started gradually by the end of 3 weeks so that by the end of 6 weeks, they are able to do all the activities including gym.
- Abdominal exercise—4 weeks
- Swimming—by 3 weeks—once the wounds are healed.

Chapter 20

Hernia in General

INTRODUCTION

More than 600,000 hernias are repaired annually in the United States, making hernia repair one of the most common operations performed by general surgeons. Despite the frequency of this procedure, no surgeon has ideal results. Complications such as postoperative pain, nerve injury, infection, and recurrence do occur.

Hernia is derived from the Latin word for rupture. It is defined as an abnormal protrusion of an organ or part of an organ through a defect in the wall of the cavity that normally contains it.[1,2] Hernias are of different kinds, based on the site, cause, contents, and symptoms, each requiring a specific management or treatment.

Although a hernia can occur at various sites of the body, these defects most commonly involve the abdominal wall, particularly the inguinal region. Abdominal wall hernias occur only at sites at which the aponeurosis and fascia are not covered by striated muscle. These sites most commonly include the inguinal, femoral, and umbilical areas; linea alba; lower portion of the semilunar line; and sites of prior incisions.

Hernia is of clinical importance because the hernial sac and its contents have the potential to become obstructed or strangulated.

Without rapid surgical intervention, the patient quickly progresses to generalized sepsis, organ failure, and death.

CLASSIFICATION OF HERNIA

Hernias can be classified according to their anatomical location as follows:

- Abdominal hernias
- Diaphragmatic hernias and hiatal hernias
- Pelvic hernias
- Lung hernias
- Muscle hernias

The most common forms of abdominal hernia, in a descending order of frequency in adults, are the inguinal (80%), epigastric (8%), incisional (7%), and femoral (5%).[3]

Each of the above hernias may be characterized by several aspects **(Box 1)**:

BOX 1: Classification of hernia.

Classification based on site:
- Groin
  - Inguinal
    - Indirect
    - Direct
    - Combined (pantaloon)
  - Femoral
  - Prevascular
- Pelvic
  - Obturator
  - Sciatic
  - Perineal
- Anterior (ventral)
  - Midline
    - Sternotomy site
    - Epigastric
    - Umbilical
    - Suprapubic
  - Lateral
    - Spigelian
    - Iliac fossa
    - Subcostal
- Posterior (lumbar)
  - Superior triangle
  - Inferior triangle
- Diaphragmatic
  - Congenital diaphragmatic hernia
  - Diaphragmatic hernia of adulthood
  - Hiatus hernia
- Internal hernias

Classification based on contents:
- Bowel
- Omentum
- Fluid
- Other
- Preperitoneal fat

Classification based on slider:
- Colon
- Bladder
- Others

Classification based on the stage of hernia:
- Reducible
- Incarcerated
- Obstructed
- Strangulated
  - Contents viable
  - Necrotic
- Perforated

Note: Also document the size of defect and whether the recurrent and other diseases are associated, such as lipoma of cord, hydrocele, and varicocele.

- *Congenital or acquired:* Congenital hernias occur prenatally or in the first year(s) of life, and are caused by a congenital defect, whereas acquired hernias develop later on in life.
- Complete or incomplete.
- *Internal or external:* External ones herniate to the outside, whereas an internal hernia does not protrude outside (e.g., hiatus hernia).
- *Intraparietal hernia:* Hernia that reaches only up to the musculoaponeurotic layer. An example is a spigelian hernia. Intraparietal hernias may produce less obvious bulging and may be less easily detected on clinical examination.
- *Bilateral:* In this case, simultaneous repair may be considered.
- *Uncomplicated or complicated:* Irreducible/strangulation/obstruction.

OTHER NAMED HERNIAS

Since many organs or parts of organs can herniate through many orifices, it is very difficult to give an exhaustive list of hernias. This book deals mostly with "visceral hernias," where the herniating tissue arises within the abdominal cavity. Other hernia types and unusual types of visceral hernias are listed as follows in an alphabetical order:

- *Amyand's hernia:* The vermiform appendix is within the hernia sac.
- *Cooper's hernia:* A femoral hernia with two sacs, the first being in the femoral canal and the second passing through a defect in the superficial fascia and appearing almost immediately beneath the skin
- *Littre's hernia:* A hernia containing Meckel's diverticulum
- *Lumbar hernia (Bleichner's hernia):* A hernia is in the lumbar region. It is of two types:
  1. *Petit's hernia:* A hernia through Petit's triangle (inferior lumbar triangle)
  2. *Grynfeltt's hernia:* A hernia through the Grynfeltt-Lesshaft triangle (superior lumbar triangle)
- *Maydl's hernia:* Two adjacent loops of small intestine are within a hernial sac with a tight neck. The intervening portion of bowel within the abdomen is deprived of its blood supply and eventually becomes necrotic.
- *Morgagni hernia:* Hernia where abdominal contents pass into the thorax through a weakness in the diaphragm
- *Pantaloon hernia (saddlebag hernia):* A combined direct and indirect hernia, when the hernial sac protrudes on either side of the inferior epigastric vessels
- *Perineal hernia:* Hernia protrudes through the muscles and fascia of the perineal floor. It may be primary, but usually is acquired following perineal prostatectomy, abdominoperineal resection of the rectum, or pelvic exenteration.
- *Properitoneal hernia:* Rare hernia located directly above the peritoneum, for example, when part of an inguinal hernia projects from the deep inguinal ring to the preperitoneal space
- *Richter's hernia:* A hernia involving only one sidewall of the bowel, which can result in bowel strangulation, leading to perforation without causing bowel obstruction
- *Sliding hernia:* It occurs when an organ drags along part of the peritoneum, or, in other words, the organ is part of the hernia sac. The colon and the urinary bladder are often involved. The term also frequently refers to sliding hernias of the stomach.
- *Sports hernia:* A hernia characterized by chronic groin pain in athletes and a dilated superficial inguinal ring
- *Velpeau hernia:* A hernia in the groin in front of the femoral blood vessels.

SIGNS AND SYMPTOMS

Hernias present with either pain at the site, a visible or palpable lump, or, in some cases, more vague symptoms resulting from pressure on an organ which has become "stuck" in the hernia, sometimes leading to organ dysfunction. Fatty tissue usually enters a hernia first, but it may be followed by an organ. The progressive clinical deterioration of a hernia can be categorized into five stages:

1. Reducible hernia
2. Irreducible hernia
3. Obstruction
4. Strangulation
5. Perforation and sepsis

Inguinal hernia is by far the most common form of abdominal hernia. It predominantly affects males, with a male:female ratio of 20:1.[3] Nevertheless, it is also the most common form of hernia seen in women.[4] It can be of direct and indirect types. In adult men, 65% of inguinal hernias are indirect.[5] Because indirect inguinal hernias run obliquely through the muscle layers within the inguinal canal, the contents of these hernias can be difficult to return to the abdominal cavity and hence are at risk of becoming strangulated. Direct inguinal hernia is uncommon in children and young adults but occurs more frequently in older people with weak abdominal musculature. In practice, both forms of hernia generally present with a lump in the groin. The affected individual may also complain of a dragging sensation in the lower abdomen, particularly when doing heavy work.

Epigastric hernia occurs in adults and arises in the linea alba. It may be small and contain only fat or become large enough to permit abdominal contents. Most small ones are asymptomatic and may be discovered incidentally as a small nodule, which is more prominent on standing. Some patients have vague upper abdominal pain similar to the pain of dyspepsia. The neck of the hernial sac is often very narrow, and because the hernia grows slowly, there is a tendency for firm scar tissue adhesions to develop between the hernial sac and its contents. Because of these two factors, almost all larger paraumbilical hernias are irreducible and hence at a high risk of obstruction and strangulation.

Incisional hernia occurs through a weak scar after a surgical operation or accidental wound. The majority of incisional hernias occur within the first 2 years of the primary operation,[6] but they can appear many years later. The first sign of an incisional hernia is usually an asymptomatic swelling over, or adjacent to, the incision site. The majority has a wide neck and does not result in obstruction or strangulation.[5] However, partial intestinal obstruction can occur in those with a narrower neck. Incisional hernia can occur as a result of open abdominal surgery or a laparoscopic procedure. Once an incisional hernia is detected, repair is usually recommended, unless other comorbid diseases pose an unacceptable risk.[6]

Femoral hernia is commonly seen in women, with a female to male ratio of 4:1.[3] It usually affects women in their 50s and 60s, particularly those who have borne children. However, male patients are more often in their 30s or 40s.[5] The right side is twice as likely to be affected as the left, but the reason for this is unknown. In 20% of cases, the hernia is bilateral. The femoral canal is very inelastic, and this leads to a high risk of strangulation. This hernia presents as strangulation in 40% of cases.[3,5,7]

Richter's hernia refers to a hernia in which only part of the circumference of the bowel gets strangulated at the neck of hernia. It occurs most commonly in femoral, obturator, and small incisional hernias.[8] As a result, intestinal obstruction is incomplete, but the bowel becomes gangrenous. Richter's hernia is most common in the sixth and seventh decades. It is responsible for 10% of cases of strangulated hernias.[9]

Obturator hernia is herniation of abdominal contents through the obturator canal. The right side is affected twice as often as the left. Obturator hernia affects women six times more commonly than men, and the majority of patients are aged over 60 years.[5] They typically occur in elderly women who have suffered a rapid loss of weight, usually due to debilitating illness. They are also more frequently seen in people of Oriental origin than in Caucasians or those of African origin.[8] Obturator hernia is rare, and difficult to diagnose, with a high proportion of cases having undergone strangulation by the time of diagnosis. The operative mortality rate approaches 30%.[8]

Gluteal and sciatic hernias are extremely rare and, like obturator hernias, are usually discovered during laparotomy to investigate the cause of a bowel obstruction.[8]

Spigelian hernia typically presents as a soft mass lateral to the rectus abdominis muscle with associated pain. It may be congenital or acquired, affecting overweight individuals, usually over 50 years of age. They also occur at the laparoscopic trocar site or even drain sites.[10]

Umbilical hernia is usually congenital, presenting as a swelling at the umbilicus in the newborn baby or young child. Failure of anatomical closure of the abdominal wall at this point results in a congenital weakness through which the hernia evolves. In most cases, this hernia is symptomless and does not require treatment, as 95% resolve spontaneously.[5] However, if the hernia remains after the age of 2 years, it requires treatment as it is then at an increased risk of strangulation. Occasionally, umbilical hernia can occur in adults, usually following pregnancy in females and in patients with chronic liver disease and ascites.

Hernias involving the diaphragm include true diaphragmatic hernias and hiatus hernias. These are different in nature from the abdominal wall hernias outlined earlier. Their symptomatology is discussed in the respective chapters.

CAUSES

The etiology of hernia is multifactorial.

- *Weakness of abdominal wall:* This may be congenital or acquired due to trauma (surgical or nonsurgical), disease, or poor body condition. Among the multiple causes, however, are the mechanical causes, which include improper heavy weightlifting, hard coughing bouts, sharp blows to the abdomen, and incorrect posture.[11] Also, if muscles are weakened due to poor nutrition, smoking, and systemic illnesses, hernias are more likely to occur.
- *Increased intra-abdominal pressure:* These include obesity, pregnancy, straining during a bowel movement or urination (constipation and enlarged prostate), chronic lung disease, and also fluid in the abdominal cavity (ascites).[12]

  Recurrence of a hernia following its initial surgical repair is a common problem. The incidence of recurrence varies from 2.3 to 20.0% for inguinal hernia and from 11.8 to 75% for femoral hernia.[13] The majority of recurrences evolve within 2–3 years of the initial repair, and these are largely due to deficiencies in the surgical technique or postoperative infection. The principal causes of recurrent hernia are outlined as follows:
  - Surgeons' experience influences the degree of tissue damage, hematoma formation, and infection.
  - *Tissues under tension:* Tissue necrosis may follow, causing breakdown of the repair and recurrence of the hernia. For this reason, the current methods of hernia repair avoid tension at the site using a prosthetic mesh.
  - Infection has been identified as a cause in around 50% of recurrent hernias. Wound infection may occur at the time of operation or postoperatively when the patient has left the hospital. The process of inflammation attracts large numbers of white blood cells, which release proteases and oxidants which destroy elastin, collagen, and other supporting structures in the tissues.[13]
  - *General condition of the patient:* Conditions such as malnutrition, low protein levels, vitamin deficiencies, jaundice, prolonged infections, chronic debilitating diseases, malignancies, and long-term steroid therapy can have a negative impact.
  - *Morbid obesity and poor nutrition:* Both lead to an increase in recurrence rates.[14]
  - *Smoking:* As explained earlier, smoking increases levels of proteases, and hence interferes with laying down collagen and wound healing. For this reason, recurrence rates are higher in smokers than nonsmokers.[15,16]

- Ascites results in increased intra-abdominal pressure. Recurrent inguinal and umbilical hernias are extremely common in patients with liver cirrhosis and ascites.
- Repeated repairs to a hernia increase the technical difficulty of the procedure, due to repeated tissue destruction and scarring. The defect increases in size with each attempt at repair and the tissues become increasingly unyielding. Large hernias typically recur more frequently than small ones.[13]
- *"Missed" hernia:* In the process of repairing an initial hernia, failure to adequately explore the inguinal and femoral canals to ensure that there are no other hernial sacs present can result in the later presentation of a hernia which appears as a "recurrence."[13]

DIAGNOSIS

Clinical examination is confirmatory in most of the cases.

Imaging [contrast-enhanced computed tomography (CECT) abdomen] is the principal means of detecting internal diaphragmatic and other nonpalpable or unsuspected hernias. It can show with precision the anatomic site of the hernia sac, the contents of the sac, and any complications.

TREATMENT

Surgery is usually recommended for most types of hernias in order to prevent complications such as obstruction of the bowel or strangulation of the tissue. The majority of patients with a groin hernia should undergo operative repair, unless they are too unfit to undergo the risks of operation. The prolonged use of trusses can be associated with complications such as atrophy of the spermatic cord and deterioration of the tissue margins of the hernial sac, and their use can make subsequent surgical repair more difficult.[16]

The surgical risks of elective hernia repair are low; therefore, few patients should be considered unfit for the procedure.[17] However, the mortality associated with strangulated inguinal and femoral hernias is high in patients who have coexistent cardiovascular or respiratory disease.[3] Surgical repair may be done by either an open operation or a laparoscopic technique. The laparoscopic approach to inguinal hernia repair is advantageous in that it results in less postoperative pain, reduced rates of persistent groin pain after a year of follow-up, and an earlier return to normal activities and work, as compared with the open operation.[3,18] The laparoscopic approach also gives the best results where the hernia is bilateral and in recurrent hernias.

REFERENCES

1. "Hernia" at Dorland's Medical Dictionary.
2. CollinsDictionary.com. Hernia. [online] Available from: https://www.collinsdictionary.com/dictionary/english/hernia [Last accessed August, 2023].

3. Cushieri A. Disorders of the abdominal wall and peritoneal cavity. In: Cushieri A, Steele RJ, Moossa AR (Eds). Essential Surgical Practice, 4th edition. London: Arnold; 2002. pp. 167-79.
4. Browse NL. An introduction to the symptoms and signs of surgical disease, 3rd edition. London: Arnold; 1997. pp. 319-38.
5. Bennett DH, Kingsnorth AN. Hernias, umbilicus, and abdominal wall. In: Russell RC, Williams NS, Bulstrode CJ (Eds). Bailey and Love's Short Practice of Surgery, 24th edition. London: Arnold; 2004. pp. 1272-93.
6. Millikan KW. Incisional hernia repair. Surg Clin North Am. 2003(83):1223-34.
7. Hachisuka T. Femoral hernia repair. Surg Clin North Am. 2003(83):1189-205.
8. Devlin HB, Kingsnorth AN. The abdominal wall and hernias. In: Burnand KG, Young AE (Eds). The new Aird's companion in surgical studies, 2nd edition. London: Churchill Livingstone; 1998. pp. 665-92.
9. Skandalakis PN, Zoras O, Skandalakis JE, Mirilas P. Richter hernia: Surgical anatomy and technique of repair. Am Surg. 2006;72(2):180-4.
10. Skandakalis PN, Zoras O, Skandakalis JE, Mirilas P. Spigelian hernia: Surgical anatomy, embryology, and technique of repair. Surg Clin North Am. 2006(72):42-8.
11. Yang XF, Liu JL. Acute incarcerated external abdominal hernia. Ann Transl Med. 2014 Nov;2(11):110. doi: 10.3978/j.issn.2305-5839.2014.11.05. PMID: 25489584; PMCID: PMC4245506.
12. Abrahamson J. Etiology and pathophysiology of primary and recurrent groin hernia formation. Surg Clin North Am. 1998(78):953-72.
13. McIntosh A, Hutchinson A, Roberts A, Withers H. Evidence-based management of groin hernia in primary care—a systematic review. Fam Pract. 2000;17(5):442-6.
14. Sugerman HJ, Kellum Jr JM, Reines HD, DeMaria EJ, Newsome HH, Lowry JW. Greater risk of incisional hernia with morbidly obese than steroid-dependent patients and low recurrence with prefascial polypropylene mesh. Am J Surg. 1996;171(1):80-4.
15. McIntosh A, Hutchinson A, Roberts A, Withers H. Evidence-based management of groin hernia in primary care—a systematic review. Fam Pract. 2000;17(5):442-7.
16. Alvarez JA, Baldonedo RF, Bear IG, Solís JAS, Alvarez P, Jorge JI. Incarcerated groin hernias in adults: Presentation and outcome. Hernia. 2004;8(2):121-6.
17. Bax T, Sheppard BC, Crass RA. Surgical options in the management of groin hernias. Am Fam Physician. 1999;59(4):893-906.
18. Nah SA, Giacomello L, Eaton S, et al. Surgical repair of incarcerated inguinal hernia in children: Laparoscopic or open? Eur J Pediatr Surg 2011;21:8–11.

Index

Page numbers followed by *f* refer to figure and *t* refer to table.

M

N

O

P